Psychoanalysis of Aging and Maturity

As developing countries increasingly confront the issues of an aging population, this important book identifies the key period in the life cycle in which changes to the body, as well as concomitant psychological developments, result in the entering of a new phase of life, maturescence.

The author defines the metapsychology of maturescence from a psychoanalytic standpoint, detaching it from the concepts of midlife and middle age. Supported by clinical examples, the book defines the stimuli which are the precursors to this phase, before examining the complete set of psychological challenges it entails. The author also highlights how maturescence has been illustrated in key literary figures in the 20th century and draws parallels with the mythical cycle of the hero.

This fascinating and original book will be essential reading for psychoanalysts, psychotherapists and any professional working with issues around aging.

Guillermo Julio Montero is a member of the International Psychoanalytical Association, President of Fundación Travesía (Psychoanalysis for Midlife Transition and Crisis), Chair of the IPA Psychoanalytic Perspectives of Aging Committee, as well as the author of several books and frequent deliverer at international psychoanalytical congresses.

"In *Psychoanalysis of Aging and Maturity: The Concept of Maturescence*, Guillermo Julio Montero offers psychoanalysis—its theory, its practitioners and its patients—a thorough and inspiring approach to the creative middle age period in the human life cycle. Through theoretical, literary and clinical considerations, he shows how the drive increase characteristic of men and women climacterics—equivalent to the one of puberty—infuses the experience of aging. The concept of *maturescence* repairs a constricted focus on 'midlife crisis' and opens our thinking to the potential for growth that the somatic and psychological transitions of middle age present."

Harriet L. Wolfe, MD, President-Elect, International Psychoanalytical Association

"In this very interesting book, Guillermo Julio Montero introduces the concept of *maturescence*, which has its roots in the Freudian idea of a universal both for women and men when they reach their 50s. From a metapsychological perspective, this universal coincides with the demand of psychic work and working through stemming from drive increase that occurs during this period of life. The way in which this psychic work is set in motion and its outcome depends on many factors, always unpredictable and singular. The author also distinguishes midlife crisis from midlife transition, both of which trigger the aging process. This book is an important contribution to the field of psychoanalysis as it shreds light into the internal processes characteristic of a period of life that has been previously studied differently."

Virginia Ungar, MD, President, International Psychoanalytical Association

Psychoanalysis of Aging and Maturity

The Concept of Maturescence

Guillermo Julio Montero

Routledge
Taylor & Francis Group

LONDON AND NEW YORK

First published 2020
by Routledge
2 Park Square, Milton Park, Abingdon, Oxon OX14 4RN

and by Routledge
52 Vanderbilt Avenue, New York, NY 10017

Routledge is an imprint of the Taylor & Francis Group, an informa business

© 2020 Guillermo Julio Montero

British Library Cataloguing-in-Publication Data
A catalogue record for this book is available from the British Library

Library of Congress Cataloging-in-Publication Data
A catalog record has been requested for this book

ISBN: 978-0-367-21837-9 (hbk)
ISBN: 978-0-367-21839-3 (pbk)
ISBN: 978-1-003-08188-3 (ebk)

Typeset in Times New Roman
by Swales & Willis, Exeter, Devon, UK

Contents

Preface

Psychoanalysis is a very strange *device*. I am suggesting this word with all the polysemy that could be assigned to the concept, since it is *something* very different from other known *somethings*. Among many other factors, psychoanalysis is strange because the transmission is carried out by other means than those in other disciplines. Consequently, psychoanalysis is not only conveyed through books, the university; its authentic transmission differs from any other (so-called) scientific *devices*.

This alien and *savage* nature of psychoanalysis is surprising because it requires making an additional effort by those who would like to practice it, having to constantly discover it. And discovering psychoanalysis is a task that those who wish to become psychoanalysts must be willing to undertake. This means that psychoanalysis *is there*; it is only a matter of discovering and owning it. Perhaps an instant will be enough, perhaps only a reflection will be sufficient … in order to possess it only for a moment. Yes, it is an evanescent *device,* and perhaps this is one of the reasons why it produces such a fascination and has the transforming power that distinguishes it.

I would therefore like to extend the use of Goethe's metaphor, so dear to Freud (1912–1913) [p. 158] 1940a [1938]) [p. 207], regarding the everyday discovery of psychoanalysis by the initiated: "What thou hast inherited from thy fathers, acquire it to make it thine" (Goethe, *Faust*, Part I, Scene I).

Freud *discovered* psychoanalysis, but the nature of the *device* forces us to rediscover it each time someone wants to start learning its art, something similar to alchemy and the work of an alchemist, if presented in this way. There is a tradition that bequeaths an inheritance, but that inheritance must be acquired, rediscovered in this case time and time again; this is psychoanalysis.

Furthermore, this does not end here because an added difficulty arises: it is impossible *to be* or *to become* psychoanalysts once and for all. With modesty, those who wish to initiate themselves in this field will only be able to remain permanently by *becoming* psychoanalysts minute by minute, day by day, a month after the previous one, etc. The present participle *becoming* allows for a liberty and spontaneity that will leave the *device* open so that it will not become obstructed by supposed truths that only lead to the cancellation of the subversive power of psychoanalysis. In this permanent becoming the work of the psychoanalyst is daily renewed; here, work acquires the equivalent status of dream *work*, symptom *work*; that is, an active process that mutates at every moment towards an objective that will satisfy a particular demand of psychic *work*.

However, psychoanalysis completes itself like a strange *device* that is very different from all others we know because it is not only *a scientific discipline* but also *a shared experience*, maintaining a complementary tension that is a excluding one at the same time. Conceived as *a scientific discipline*, it can be measured, validated as well as refuted; whereas as *a shared experience* it is nontransferable, impossible to translate, codify and transmit in a reliable manner outside the experience itself. Therefore, from the perspective of *a scientific discipline*, parameters can be used that validate it only with a measurement that is undertaken off-line: here the key—*ultima ratio* as well as *primum movens*—is psychoanalytic metapsychology; whereas, from the perspective of *a shared experience*, it becomes impossible—also absolutely unnecessary if it were possible—to steer a scientific determination of the experience itself, since a claim of this sort being on-line—immersed in the situation—would totally invalidate the psychoanalytic process, thus raising the philosophical problem of knowledge that gnoseology has attempted to unsuccessfully decipher for centuries.

From this standpoint, there would be no need to force an exclusive inclusion within the so-called *scientific field*, since psychoanalysis is something which implies such a special vertex that it has the advantage of being able to validate itself by itself. If the supposition that the experience and intimacy shared in the consulting room is valuable only if the so-called scientific parameters could be measured, where would this lead?

In this regard, sometimes psychoanalysis would seem to suffer from a kind of *inferiority complex* with respect to other fields. This would explain why it would want to be included among other scientific fields at all costs, forgetting in this way the transcendental *handcrafted* effort an *authentic* psychoanalytic treatment implies, which is beyond any kind of reliable measurement ... fortunately for everybody: patients and psychoanalysts. This so happens because it is a human experience more than a laboratory test and perhaps for this reason there is no need to replicate and evaluate it with variables that are alien to the very nature of psychoanalysis.

Possibly, the demand for scientific validation does not arise so much from psychoanalysis itself but rather from the widespread psychoanalytically based psychotherapy. Perhaps the triangulation suggested by psychotherapeutic treatments with the inclusion of the health system or health insurance as a *third party* included in the phantasmatic scene shared by both patient and psychotherapist—often forcing a difficult transferential elaboration in order to clear up the analytic field—makes it necessary to acknowledge psychoanalysis as a science.

If scientific validation were an essential requisite, it is important then to distinguish between psychotherapy and psychoanalysis, thus ending the dispute. Psychoanalysis would then have the *freedom of action* to achieve its purpose of gaining access to the unconscious truth, something which does not need to be confirmed except in the analytic setting, in the transference, in the intimacy of the consulting room. Here two paths seem to diverge between "the pure gold of analysis" and "the copper of direct suggestion" (psychotherapy?), in Freud's words (1919a [1918]) [p. 168].

For these reasons, I would not be pleased if psychoanalysis became scientific, in which case it would run the risk of becoming *pasteurized* instead of maintaining the *contaminated*, *subversive*, *savage* and *untamed* validity that carries human desires and wishes—the mark in the selvedge bequeathed by Freud more than one hundred years ago.

This way of thinking does not pretend to condemn psychotherapy to uselessness: on the contrary. Generally the patient seeks psychotherapy and not psychoanalysis; the latter cannot and usually is not an *a priori*; it is also a resource that can be reached as the result of an achievement in psychotherapy. The patient seeks help because he experiments anxiety, and the psychoanalyst suggests a *device* that hopes to solve it: from then on the path to psychoanalysis can be opened.

This same formulation of the tension between the *laboratory* and the *experience* becomes valid for the so-called *specialty areas*. A book like the one the reader is holding does not pretend to be a treaty on maturescence and its derivatives—midlife, middle age, beginning of aging, etc.—in order to propose a certain *specialty area* of the topic. Nothing could be further from my intention.

My idea is that it is essential to understand the metapsychology underlying the maturescent experience, which must always be considered off-line since, only immersed in the psychoanalytic process is it possible to treat the internal universe of a particular and unique individual; something quite different from a person who is aging or aged.

The proposal implies considering the metapsychological study of maturescence in order to *forget it* or *set it aside* at the precise instant the psychoanalyst closes the door of his consulting room to share the psychoanalytic experience with the patient—moment from which metapsychology operates from a background where it would seem to constitute itself in the silent continent that facilitates and contains the content of the whole experience—regardless of whether the patient is undergoing maturescence or any other moment of the vital cycle. This guarantees a certain authenticity to the whole process of psychoanalysis because suggesting *applied* psychoanalysis to someone who is aging or someone who has already aged can only result in a psychoanalytic *as if*, with a time-worn, false and inauthentic result, a *pasteurized* outcome, perhaps innocuous, as previously stated.

True applied psychoanalysis has a different aim: to comprehend a work of art, whether a novel, a film, a play, a painting, etc., being absolutely relevant and valid in the situations noted, but with the great difference of knowing that one is operating *per via di porre* (mass-produced), instead of *per via di levare* (tailor-made), as Leonardo da Vinci and Freud (1904a [1904], p. 260) said. The risk of *applying* psychoanalysis to the maturescent patient would lead to running the parallel risk that the psychoanalytic process be marred by contaminating itself with previous concepts that can hinder the psychoanalyst's liberty to listen, by operating *per via di porre*, instead of *per via di levare*.

Of course, this is also valid for all the so-called *specialty areas*: childhood, adolescence, addictions, depressions, etc. *Applying* psychoanalysis may become iatrogenic because it inevitably sets aside the subjectivity of the patient if the listening is predetermined by concepts that clog up the essential liberty *to be there*. For this reason, I highlight a perspective centered on subjectivity—from inside out—instead of doing it from the opposite perspective—from outside in.

I know that a book like this one runs the risk of turning into an *introductory handbook* on maturescence. I would like to point out that I distrust *handbooks* for various reasons. They tend to function as authentic inhibitors of autonomous thinking. For this reason, these words would like to avoid falling into frequently incurred generalizations. This book only aims at being useful to understand the metapsychology of maturescence—that latter being the theoretic *princeps device* that allows the psychoanalyst to infer interpretations during the session; it is a tool that the therapist already has internalized long before.

Perhaps due to the difficulty of referring to *shared experiences*, the reader will find few clinical examples of psychoanalytic treatments—the interpretation of a patient's dream, two interpretations of the maturescent processing in two patients, not more—and many examples linked to classical and contemporary literature. On the other hand, I believe that the *applied* examples are definitely valuable to transmit an authentic experience because the reader has the same resources owned by the psychoanalyst that interprets them: in this case, the rules of the game are clear because there are no disguised data.

In conclusion, the task is twofold: the work that involves *discovering* psychoanalysis and the work of *becoming* a psychoanalyst. The tension between these two tendencies is what gives authentic life to the search of each *initiated* therapist who, in his efforts, will follow a path that will obtain different results—investigations, papers, books, lectures—that will evince not only the task of *discovering* psychoanalysis once again, but the task of *becoming* a psychoanalyst. I would like the reader to consider that, of course, the metapsychology of maturescence presented here is the result of my own attempt not only *to discover* psychoanalysis but also *to become* a psychoanalyst every day of my life.

The reader will find in this book a personal work, unusual in some respects because the state-of-the-art, among other things, appears as the last chapter. The reason lies in the fact that when I started to research what had been written about middle age, I came upon several books and papers that described the phenomenon from very different perspectives; in many cases, with post-Freudian visions. Several years later, I began to discover by myself that which I was beginning to understand through my maturescent patients, could also be inferred in Freud's work. For this reason, I dedicated my efforts to delve into this process.

The attempt to describe the metapsychology of maturescence from the perspective of Freud's work offers an important advantage: Freud's work is our mother tongue. That is the reason why it is necessary to share the root experience of this effort in the first place. Only afterwards the post-Freudian tenets, also important, begin to have any value. The motto for my proposal regarding maturescence, therefore, is: "Instead of returning to Freud, I propose depart from Freud." And it is from this positioning that all subsequent developments acquire any meaning.

The effort to coin a new concept may also seem to contradict what I have set forth in the previous paragraphs. The idea of *maturescence*, however, implies the consideration of a specific moment—something synchronic—in contrast to the decades that can be considered as middle age—something diachronic. Similarly, the concept of *midlife*—despite sounding both synchronic and diachronic—is inappropriate because it became associated with the representation of midlife crisis, an insufficient concept to account for that which characterizes the specialty and totality of maturescent processing, as it will be explained in the following chapters. For this reason, I consider legitimate to introduce *the concept of maturescence* in order to define it from Freudian concepts, as I hope will be clearly set out in this book.

Acknowledgements

Thanking all those who have been part of my psychoanalytic education and training is not an easy matter. I am sure that by naming just a few and forgetting many others I will commit an injustice.

Nevertheless, if I had to make a summary, I am grateful to Calvin Anthony Colarusso MD (San Diego, California, US), whose human warmth permitted a daily communication based on our scientific interests: we edited and published papers, presented symposiums in congresses, without forgetting to talk about life and trying to live it; all this simply after I made contact with him because I was interested in his works until time did its work, making possible for our friendship to extend itself to family ties that honor me with the authenticity and sincerity that have remained firm throughout all these years.

In addition, I would like to thank Virginia Ungar MD (Buenos Aires, Argentina) for her cordiality and great human qualities, always ready to promote and facilitate new horizons, receiving proposals with a warm smile and making it possible to turn them into reality.

I would also like to thank Rubén Mario Basili MD (1935–1917) (Buenos Aires, Argentina) for his generosity for jointly sharing so many friendly hours and a lot of papers.

I would also like to thank my colleagues at the International Psychoanalytical Association's Committee: *Psychoanalytic Perspectives on Aging*, of which I am honored to be its Chair and with whom I have established a sincere friendship as well as the wish to make known our way of understanding aging. This has led to the production of important work that continues up to now. Its members are: Audrey Kavka (United States), Valeria Egidi Morpurgo (Italy; who died in 2009, sadly), María Cristina Reis Amendoeira (Brazil), Mi Yu (United States), Daniel Plotkin (United States), Renata Sgier (Switzerland), Gianina Micu (Romania), and Alex Oxenberg (Chile).

Finally, I would like to thank my translator, Ms Maria Squirru, for the dedication and commitment with which she undertook the project of translating this book. As always, I have reserved the last word for the final edition. Consequently, should any errors have slipped by, I own up to them.

Further acknowledgements

To my wife, my love, and life companion Alicia: thank you for being there, always the same and always different.

To my children Nicolás, Leopoldo and Julián; I still see them grow while I age: a beautiful paradox.

To their partners María, Daniela and Victoria, who not only share complicities in each encounter but also life-in-itself.

To my grand-daughter Pia, who has the privilege of being the first—for now.

To my nephew Manuel, a true dreamer of the future, together with Gisela, Graciela and Claudio.

To my dear friend Ignacio, schemer of impossible ventures.

To María Gloria, who shares the love for research.

To Betty, Fernando, and María de los Ángeles.

To my friends Pablo and María, mutual confidants of many projects that we are sure will come to fruition.

To my colleagues and friends at the Travesía Foundation, with whom we have shared the dream of growing together for the past thirty years.

To my colleagues from the Doctorate Program, with whom we enjoyed several challenging years.

To my colleagues and friends of the Argentine Psychoanalytic Association.

To my patients, who tolerate all that I cannot manage to truly comprehend.

To all those whom I am forgetting.

All of them.

Glossary

Maturescence
: The psychic outcome to the true beginning of biological aging. It is fostered and shaped through a universal drive increase which Freud already linked to somatic climacterics phenomena in men and women. Each individual will work through these exigencies of psychic work with his/her own psychic resources, allowing the selection and manifestation of a series of paths depicting different subjective landscapes, procedures and aims.

Maturity
: The end result of maturescent working-through and midlife symptomatic manifestations during middle age, ending with the subjective perception of a greater psychic space and a renewed experience with time, something that makes reality become more lifelike through the enhancing and deepening of individual identity.

Midlife
: The symptomatic manifestations of maturescence depicting a series of different subjective landscapes, procedures and aims which encompass a continuum between the extreme poles of midlife transition and midlife crisis. Each individual will traverse it in his/her own way, trying to find a renewed tension and bond between the pleasure principle and the reality principle, something that maturescent drive increase not only challenges but threatens to split.

Middle age
: A period of years ranging between age forty-five to age sixty-five beginning with maturescence and ending with old age and ensuing senescence. There are no previous universal psychological tasks or frames to go through, but really different individual needs and wishes to be tamed, promoted and fulfilled in order to guarantee the living continuity and achievement of psychic growth and inner development.

Chapter I

Mid-life

Steps to be taken before the introduction of a new concept

The 1960s decade was paradigmatic because it was a time when many Western youngsters began to occupy a transcendental place that was different in the human vital cycle—a vital spot which had never been previously filled. From that moment on it was possible to define youth as an important stage of life with its own identity and subjectivity. This was not the result of any particular concession; on the contrary, it was the determination of making a commitment with their lives that perhaps attempted to avoid some of the phantoms and fears brought by the Second World War, long after it ended. The phenomenon can be understood as a reaction to the failure of a generation that led the world to such a manifested disaster: a way of self-defense, a desire of giving birth to something that was different to what their parents had endured. Furthermore, the sixties' revolution can be conceived as a way of self-protection against an adult world that had sent a lot of young people to die in the Vietnam War.

These youths—as a generation—began to have their own voice, which demanded to be heard. Young people were convinced that they had something to say and this was an unprecedented phenomenon. The concept of an oncoming social revolution that would change the world order, the idea that a new man existed who had to be discovered, the possibility of investing in a future with a notion of renovated liberty, were premises that erupted in the public stage with unusual force, unknown until then. And this occurred simultaneously throughout the Western world as a synchronic phenomenon—an emerging *global village* before information technology (IT) developed its own revolution, transforming the world in an authentic global village. In fact, it had already been suggested by Marshall McLuhan (1962)—something that today remains sounding prophetic as well as anticipatory of a future of hyper-connectivity at all levels, anticipated by the available media of those days; innocent devices, compared to the ones available nowadays. Perhaps McLuhan never dreamt that his theory would become such a notorious reality as it actually turned out to be; neither did his followers and exegetes, but it all came to pass.

Important cities of the Western world were filled with young demonstrators who took to the streets demanding, confronting and affirming that they would never adopt the hypocritical and mediocre attitude received as their parents' legacy; the latter had failed and therefore they would change the world forever. The youngsters' motto, "Don't trust anyone over thirty," became famous and was repeated like a mantra during those years, serving as a rite of passage both in Europe and the United States. A similar phenomenon took place in Latin America, although the political situation was totally different to the one in the northern hemisphere. Each region had its own way of expressing itself within a context of discontent and desire for self-assertion.

The student revolt that took place in France in May, in 1968, the struggle against the war in Vietnam and the libertarian and anti-establishment movements that occurred in the United States (hippies, flower power, pacifism, situationism, surrealism, mysticism, Buddhism, experience with drugs, etc.), the Cuban revolution and guerrilla movements in Latin America, the sexual revolution, the appearance of new musical expressions—from the most well-known musical groups to the possibility of individuals experimenting the new music at home, connected by electricity, from massive rock shows to private ones held by musical elites of experimental jazz—are just some of the examples of the need for identification shared by thousands of youths, all with the aim of changing the world as it was known up to then.

Perhaps the poets of the Beat Generation in San Francisco, led by Lawrence Ferlinghetti as editor and Allen Ginsberg as the iconic messianic figure, who proposed a *Howl* against Society in ceremonies and street shows, were the authentic forerunners during the fifties of the youth movement of the subsequent decade; they had already fought against all types of prejudices, welcoming blacks, jews, drug addicts, homosexuals, communists and anarchists to their movement.

Nothing indicated in the sixties that in the midst of the youth revolution the concept of mid-life crisis—related to another very different stage of life—would appear with such overwhelming force; none the less it did. The pioneering work *Death and the Mid-Life Crisis* by Elliott Jaques was published in the *The International Journal of Psycho-Analysis* in 1965, producing its own revolution; it was a concept that was there to stay.

In some way, the concept of a mid-life crisis functioned as a cultural reaction of the adult generation to the attacks of the youth of that time so as to re-delineate adult identity, something that was becoming blurred, overrode and somehow debased.

From *mid-life crisis* to the uncanny and universal *midlife crisis*

The concept of *mid-life crisis* was fully accepted by psychoanalysts from its very beginning when it was proposed by Jaques (1965). This is not the place to debate if he was right—or whether this author agrees with Jaques' ideas or not—but he was wise enough to give a Kleinian and useful background to a psychological phenomenon. So far, everything is normal: a new and success-ful concept within the psychoanalytic framework in the midst of a changing world.

Can we think of the success of the concept as a reaction by the adult world—in this case—with respect to youths that endeavoured to acquire a precise identity in the life cycle, almost for the first time in history?

Be it as it may, something strange happened with the idea of *mid-life crisis* because the concept immediately popped out from its psychoanalytic origin and spread throughout society—something rather uncommon. Popular culture made the rest, adopting it as one of its dearest ideas: films, novels, soap operas, cartoons, jokes, a lot of popular and artistic creations and media con-tents made the concept theirs:

How can this be explained?
Why did it occur and why is it still happening?

We may think that the disturbing evidence of something really special happen-ing during *mid-life crisis* worked not only as a sociological and anthropological answer but also as a psychoanalytic interpretation and insight, and led society to appropriate this concept as the expression and natural way out of an *uncanny* evidence of the shadow of unconscious feelings that dwell within us. And here the word *uncanny* is the proper one because it places strangeness in the ordinary world—something oddly familiar rather than simply mysterious, as; Freud (1919h) [p. 219] states.

But this *uncanny* feeling is not enough to make the concept of *mid-life crisis* so popular. The power of the concept not only comes from its *uncanny* roots: it is enhanced and stressed due to its universality: everybody goes under an equivalent psychic state of mind at a certain age in the life cycle.

More, the concept of mid-life crisis continues moving us in the same way that Greek tragedy does, created more than two thousand years ago. In the case of Greek tragedy, it is because of its universality: certain human conflicts have not changed; otherwise, they would have been played and enjoyed at the moment but immediately forgotten. From this vertex, *mid-life crisis* succeeded as a popular concept because of its twofold constitution: not only an uncanny feeling but also its universality are its components.

This author believes that the power and pregnancy of the concept of *mid-life crisis* comes from the inner and mysterious uncanny place where all human beings remain tied to biology—as if they were powerful minds trying to over-whelm and defeat the power of biology and its mandate, instead of assuming their humble and transient bodies, trying to find a meaning to nonsense while life lasts.

Up to this moment, the concept of *mid-life* remains tied to the concept of *crisis* as if they were just one—and they remain linked as if they were one from the beginning.

Why does this occur?

What is the *crisis* of *mid-life*?

What would have happened if Jaques' concept were just *mid-life* or if he would have dealt only with *mid-life*?

Possibly, nothing would have happened and perhaps the concept would have been forgotten. *Mid-life* is a stage of life—of course, a long and universal one—but it lacks the *uncanny* content of *crisis*—another universal. Both universals are needed to give the concept its power. From this perspective, *crisis* may be the proper qualifying adjective for *mid-life*.

What does *crisis* mean?

Is *crisis* the needed universal component for *mid-life*?

It may be thought that *crisis* has a strong effect on the expression *mid-life crisis* because this qualifying factor is something that makes evident the enormous amount of psychic work demanded by specific unconscious feelings. Summarizing: *mid-life* is posed as a stage of life—a long period of years—and *mid-life crisis* may be understood as the beginning of this stage of life called *mid-life*—up to that moment commonly known as *middle age*—such a common word as to discard the hyphen and simply consider it as *midlife*.

A historical perspective on the concept of midlife crisis

In retrospect, the success of the concept could be related to an adult reaction to the youth movement of those days. Almost as if adult identity could have rebelled against the power that the youth movement pretended to sustain or really did possess at the time. In other words, this adult identity manifested itself like a reactive formation, maintaining an identitary affirmation in the midst of so much discredit to adulthood per se. In this way, not only the young reinforced their generational identity but so did the new so-called midlifers.

Some data can evince this phenomenon a bit better. For example, Google's N-Gram browsing tool, after digitalizing millions of books published between 1800 and 2010, show a trend with a certain degree of validity. The N-Grams demonstrate the frequency with which a word appears in books—newspapers, magazines are not included—that were being edited, without discriminating between scientific production and dissemination production. This may indicate the importance of a word as social representation or its presence in the collective worldview.

The search with the expression *midlife crisis* or *mid-life crisis* confirms the affirmation of an irruption of the concept: it makes its appearance during the mid-1960s—without any mention prior to that date—showing a sharp rising curve in the number of mentions which is surprising. It should be noted that the result is the same if only the word *midlife* (without hyphen) is considered.

Moreover, the mid-life crisis concept did not just function as a reaction but as a kind of psychoanalytic interpretation as well, in a manner equivalent to how interpretation functions in psychoanalysis, since it affected the understanding of the life cycle in a manner unknown until then. An interpretation decentralizes: it operates a change and allows for a new understanding of a phenomenon. This is precisely what occurred with Jaques' pioneering concept and work because it immediately became part of popular culture—newspapers, literary works and plays, scientific works, etc.—as already anticipated, perhaps leading to the assumption that everyone would undergo what was beginning to be identically termed as midlife crisis.

It can undoubtedly be sustained that the midlife crisis is a universal. However, one of the purposes of this book is to make evident that it is not possible to determine the value of a psychic phenomenon by its external semiology. On the contrary, it must be done by also using a metapsychology that can evince the specific working-through processes—not necessarily inferable by the conduct. For this reason, many of the efforts made to understand the midlife crisis only linked the manifested content of the conduct with a stereotype. This led to the erroneous assumption that everyone had to undergo the midlife crisis in a similar way.

In order to illustrate this point, we could consider that a person is experiencing a creative process every time he or she paints a picture or writes a poem. From this perspective, the manifested behavior could lead to an error because the result of the creative experience—*experience* is a significant word that will be examined in a later chapter—cannot be assessed only by the supposedly created artistic product but rather by the inner psychic processing that the individual experiences during the creative process. A great external similarity exists between a creative process and an evacuative process, as well as a huge intra-psychic difference. Both processes can only be distinguished by means of a metapsychological understanding—an exclusive territory of psychoanalysis—since the latter makes it possible to distinguish both types of psychic processes. Psychoanalytically speaking, if the perspective of internal processing is not considered, it is impossible to say a word about the authentic provenance of one or the other of these extreme vertexes.

From this perspective, therefore, it is possible to affirm that the midlife crisis is a universal, but a universal that is psychically processed by the individual according to the availability of the psychic working-through of each one, taking into account processing possibilities that are always completely different because they depend on complementary series, prevailing defensive mechanisms, different conflict situations, etc.

However, considering the midlife crisis as a universal implies an authentic definition and characterization of this universal:

What are we referring to when we sustain this universal?
What universal is the word universal referring to?

All this will be dealt with in the following chapter.

But—returning to the function of midlife crisis as interpretation—in order for an interpretation to produce a change, a need for that change is always necessary beforehand. The interpretation must coincide with that which the individual intimately hopes will happen—even though he or she might not initially recognize it as his or her own. We could maintain, therefore, that the concept midlife crisis existed in a latent state in society, a kind of Bionian pre-conception that Jaques was able to conceptualize—almost in the manner of an interpretation. This is why it lasted and started to represent a phenomenon that expanded rapidly with a value of its own. From then on, an exegetical effort commenced in order to have access to its authentic meaning, giving rise to a great quantity of books and papers that referred to the topic.

So many efforts in defining the concept perhaps led to a certain darkness of representations, reason why many times what Jaques termed *mid-life crisis* can be confused with *middle age*—confusing a specific moment with a more extended period, as has already been anticipated.

Some characteristics and factors of the midlife crisis

Various authors maintain that the midlife crisis—*midlife crisis* as a general concept in this case—can promote a greater wisdom (Erikson, 1951), an increment or transformation of one's creativity (Jaques, 1965), the possibility of enjoying a renewed intimacy (Neugarten, 1996), a better use of one's time (Colarusso, 1999), and many other factors and characteristics.

Perhaps it would be appropriate to consider that these *characteristics* can be the result of a successful passage through the midlife crisis, but this is not always the case. On the contrary, the typical outcome—*typical* understood as the more popular social representation of the phenomenon—of the midlife crisis would imply the exact opposite: confusion, perplexity, uncertainty, acting-out, depression, etc. In view of these affirmations, several questions may be raised:

> What causes this to occur?
> What authentic device is set in motion?
> How, when and for what reason can the result imply a successful course—*psychologically* successful, in the sense of the individual's satisfaction—and when and why can the result of the course and destiny turn out to be different?
> What really happens?

In several cases we could suppose that those characteristics were fulfilled by simply getting through that specific moment of the life cycle and undoubtedly this is so, but we should point out that they are not universal destinies and characteristics; it is not sufficient to reach a certain age in order to acquire them. These characteristics describe something that does not happen to everyone but rather to a few people, under certain internal circumstances.

Following this train of thought, a deconstruction of the concept of midlife crisis becomes necessary—in line with the forthcoming proposition regarding *maturescence*, main target of this book—commencing with an effort to remove the shadows that obscure the perspective of an authentic psychic processing, in order to subsequently propose a renovated mode of comprehension.

But in order to answer the questions just formulated, the authors whom we previously made reference to propose that the special changes that appear at this period of life could be the consequence of certain *factors*—so named to distinguish them from the *characteristics* already alluded to—such as: the empty nest syndrome (when the children leave home); facing illness, aging or death of their own parents; the eventual illness or death of a close friend; that the individual might be going through some complex illness, perhaps incurable, just to name a few. The *factors* may be numerous, but they can all result in an indirect comprehension or prejudice.

These assumptions would suggest a way of acquiring these *characteristics* which would allow for the enjoyment of a new stage in adult life, but only by overcoming some experiences of mourning. The ideas put forward refer precisely to the processing of mourning that can occur normally and naturally during the middle age of most people, although not necessarily everyone.

But more would follow because, if these are the *factors* that would help to promote the changes suggested, we must consider the huge contradiction that they are not universal phenomena. Perhaps someone did not have children and will not, therefore, have to face the mentioned elaboration. The same thing occurs with the second example: it could be that the individual lost his parents when they were very young and never really knew them; this kind of grieving, therefore, would not be experienced. It could also happen that none of his friends would become sick or die during this period, and that the person himself was in good health. Would this mean that we would be barred from access to the wisdom of life, from creativity, from a different intimacy, or a renovated way of internally experiencing time? The answer, obviously, is that those experiences are also possible to someone who did not go through some or any of the mentioned situations.

Perhaps underlying this kind of reasoning there is a motive that could be interpreted as sustaining that pain facilitates personal growth and only those who have suffered some kind of loss are able to acquire that special *something* that middle age has to offer. However, it is very difficult to subscribe to a proposition of this nature because it would work as a common ground— the "common ground" as a relative of "common sense," as will be discussed later in this book—that maintains that a person values health only when he loses it, but this idea would work best as an example of neurosis than of possible growth. Perhaps this is true only for those who need to manage their inner selves with these types of threats in order to attempt some inner growth, necessarily false if the starting point is not genuine, as the one detailed through a state where what is at stake is the urgency of recuperating something that has been lost:

> How could it be possible to consider that something like this could imply an authentic personal growth?

If it is necessary to lose something in order to value it and thus acquire a compensation, we would then be in the presence of a reactive device—obviously impoverishing—totally unrelated to psychic development. Perhaps, underlying this kind of reasoning, some (falsely) religious ideas are being hidden; namely, human beings are meant to suffer and we will therefore find eternal happiness in a different life, subsequent to the mandatory levy that would have to be paid with suffering—such as this example sustains.

This is so because that which is acquired reactively (perhaps from a regressive perspective?) can be qualitatively differentiated from something generated with a proactive aim (from a progressive perspective, perhaps?), since this is the perspective from which any psychic phenomenon linked to psychic development can be psychoanalytically understood.

A good example of this situation could be found in the management of physical health. It is not recommended that a person should eat healthily in order not to get sick, but rather to be well: healthy, strong, balanced, simply because this is as it should be by nature. Personal care is an essential condition—never an exception derived from any other problem or dysfunction. Once that personal care is lost, a deteriorating process commences that may seem invisible at first, but that slowly begins to give its first signals. The regressive (reactive) position in this case would be the desperate attempt to recuperate something that was lost, whereas the progressive (proactive) position would imply maintaining a disposition that has to be naturally present.

This is a fine example to make visible what is derived from the (false) religious position—human beings would suffer on earth but will be rewarded in the afterlife—linked to the concept that losses are useful or help growth: it is not necessary, neither is it valuable or useful—to lose something in order to value it. When this occurs, it makes evident that other situations already exist that evince the loss of direction. The "natural" attitude—with all the resonance the word will have in this book—is progressive—and not regressive, something which implies a qualitative vertex that is totally different.

These considerations led to the need of defining more precisely what and how really happens in what was called midlife crisis.

For an understanding of *maturescence*

The proposal of the midlife crisis which we have made reference to is an attempt to lay the path that will permit the development of the hypothesis of *maturescence*, the underlying psychic process that could be considered as a universal.

It is evident for this author that another factor exists, powerful but noiseless, which is universal and has been common to men and women throughout history, regardless of individual differences—nationality, race, geographic location. The *characteristics* (wisdom, creativity, intimacy, reassessment of time, etc.) and the *factors* (empty nest syndrome, illness and/or death of parents, illness and death of peers, serious illness of the individual himself, etc.) are events which, raised in this manner, seem completely uprooted from the *actual experience* (with all the signification this concept has for psychoanalysis) that each person is experiencing. Explicitly put: it is not enough as a valid explanation to take one of these *factors* to justify a whole period of one's life—to take a part for the whole. In order to make an appropriate theorization, it is essential to consider the authentic provenance of the phenomena that characterize a period or stage of life.

Science has a certain obligation to theorize universal phenomena. Otherwise, the conclusions to which it arrives cannot be generalized. The purpose of this book is to contribute to the understanding of maturescence arising from a universal factor, remaining open to all individual differences, be they positive or negative, creative or destructive, transcendental or intranscendental. In other words, an anchor point from where all individual variations are possible.

To clarify these ideas, perhaps we could use the metaphor of the construction and flight of a kite which, in order to fly high needs a supportive point with feet well grounded; if this were not so, and the kite was released, it would fall to the ground, following an unpredictable path. The same would occur if the kite string snapped due to the tension provoked by a strong wind: it would fall in a matter of seconds. But, whatever the case might be, the kite could never rise and display its full potential without a firm anchor point—the thumb and index fingers holding the string, the act of slowly letting go of the string so that it could reach the greatest height, etc. Nevertheless, it could fly high or low, displaying with the breeze the colors selected by its maker, the place and time of day selected—these are the individual variations or choices selected by the individual who decides to make the kite fly.

The concept of maturescence developed in this book is presented as a universal factor that allows for a universal anchorage point and a high degree of individual variability—without prejudices—which permits "flying" towards many different individual destinies. This proposal is in stark contrast with those who suggest that there are *factors* that activate a kind of processing that derives in uniform *characteristics* during the course of midlife. The following pages, therefore, will attempt to refute the latter proposal.

The acknowledgement of reality

With the sort of explanations that refer to *factors* and *characteristics*, something similar to Plato's allegory of the cave would be occurring; an excellent metaphor that illustrates how false knowledge can be confused with true knowledge. In the mentioned allegory, the causes and effects seem to appear interchanged, in which case certain illusory manifestations are similar to mirages that decentralize the true comprehension of the problem's origin, making it confusing.

Let us analyze Plato's proposition, as it appears in *The Republic*. A group of prisoners are chained by their necks and legs to a wall. They are forced to look at the wall in front of them, unable to look backwards or sideways. They can only see a series of shadows projected on the wall, which they are forced to take as real; in fact, it is the only reality they have ever known. The shadows are projected by men who are hidden from the prisoners' view. They transport banners with whose forms are projected by the light of a fire which is behind the prisoners. The latter, in turn, attribute what they see as real because they cannot perceive it in any other way; if they could get up and walk, for example, they would discover the ploy. The men decide that one of the prisoners may be conducted to the knowledge of reality and therefore set him free. When the freed prisoner returns with the news that a different world lies outside the cave, he is murdered by his previous fellow captives, who cannot give credence to what their former companion says.

Even though the allegory of the cave may be useful and lend itself to multiple interpretations, philosophic, anthropological, epistemological, among others—and could even be understood as a hidden model for the discovery of the Freudian model of interpretation of dreams—it serves in this case as a paradigmatic example of how appearances can hide authentic reality, diverting us from a true understanding of phenomena; in other words, how it is possible to be deceived taking for truth what is not so. Albeit Plato's purpose would seem to be pedagogic, the allegory also demonstrates how simple it is to divert one's attention towards that which appears as an effect—appearances, if we follow the allegory—rather than towards the causes—the true basis and fundamental purpose of all things.

We may think that what is proposed as the cause (*factors*) of certain phenomena (*characteristics*) of the midlife crisis has little to do with the origin or true causes that originate the mentioned specificity; neither are they related to the alluded consequences, since they are not universals, but neither do they stem from the alluded causes.

In that case, the conditions are worse than that of the prisoners in the cave because the latter have been deceived from what is real truth. If they dared discover the intent, they would understand the deceit. In the case of the *factors* and *characteristics*, however, it would be worse because what seems true and real in fact is not; or perhaps it is real but only from the point of view of certain consequences, which are not universals either. Sustaining the validity and theoretical usefulness of *factors* and *characteristics* would be worse than confusing appearance with reality—something very much in line with the allegory of the cave.

For this reason a universal factor is suggested, encompassing both men and women, which facilitates an explanation—it would be like the authentic fire behind the prisoners that tricks them into assuming as real what in fact is not so, thus accepting the shadows projected by those who want to deceive them regarding the nature of reality.

The universal factor suggested is intimately linked to human *nature*. We would like to make clear that the word *nature* is written in its true sense: human nature alludes to the *biological nature* of human beings.

It should be noted that when we refer to human beings, they are to be understood as one of the species, not as a different thing, not as a kind of a non-species, despite the huge difference between us and the rest of the species. The human species is only one among millions of others that inhabit the planet. The cornerstone of our humanity has its roots in our *biological nature*; human beings are conditioned by nature, no matter how much this has been denied.

Human beings struggle to deny being part of nature with everything that lies in their power. This accounts for many of the serious problems that humanity endures: that which is based on a negation or a denial has no possibility of flowing appropriately towards resolutions aimed at an authentic common good or joint community effort. Perhaps due to this negation and denial, the human species is the only one where such strange events like mass inter-species killings occur; of course, we do not leave out all the positive aspects of the human species which distinguish it from the rest but we shall return to this point later on.

The cause of the events that promote what has been termed the great change that occurs at middle age—both those considered favorable as well as those that are not—has to do with a fact that it is part of nature and implies, therefore, a universal biological mark: masculine and feminine climacterics. This period of life fulfills the role of the fire in Plato's allegory of the cavern: the fire makes the shadow projections possible producing true effects, albeit always hiding its origin.

Climacterics in human beings, although experienced by all species, has a distinguishing feature with respect to other species—perhaps it is a significant factor—because the human species is the only one that after menopause in women, and after the diminution or cessation of men's fertile period, endeavors to go on living as long as possible. Most known superior species die soon after the commencement of infertility. In this respect, we could consider life after climacterics as a human "invention."

It is hard to understand when and how this effort to maintain ourselves alive, at whatever cost, began. It is not easy to provide an explanation but perhaps the emergence of language, or the possibility of "representing" reality, by means of the human brain, no matter how incipient this language might have been at first, is what marked this difference.

The biologist Jared Diamond (1992) refers to a "great leap forward"; a mythical moment when what differentiates us from other species took place. And despite the fact that we share 98% of our genetic code with superior apes, that remaining 2% is what distinguishes us from them. Moreover it is argued that language was what brought about this great difference rather than the acquisition of conscience. Even though it is not easy to suppose that conscience preceded language or vice versa, it is believed that a form of rudimentary language began to be shared in daily interaction, which could have led to language itself, rudimentary as it might have been.

Long before Diamond, Freud (1915a) presented an answer, even though he was not trying to answer the question just posed. According to Freud, this occurred at a mythical moment in the evolutionary history of humanity when human beings began to represent their instinctive lives; in other words, when we became conscious of our biological nature, by representing it. Without going into details, Freud suggested that our instinctive nature could begin to be represented in an order of discourse, which is why we could propose here the *great leap forward*, so well defined metaphorically by Diamond, from the perspective of psychoanalysis.

However, what is important in order to understand the distinguishing 2% of the genetic code that differentiates humans from superior apes is that the human species gave a huge step forward when it gained access to language as a way of representation of itself and the world; especially with regard to its own finitude.

The awareness of death would seem to be absent in other species, despite the enormous effort made by a simple insect attempting to escape from mortal danger. It is difficult to determine what value we could give to what many biologists term flight reflex. These affirmations could belie the idea that human beings are unique and the top of the evolutionary scale; a further disguise of some religious ideas that explain the origin of the world and of life in an absolutist manner.

Be this as it may, before and after climacterics, the human species tries to survive as much as it can. Science spends huge amounts of money to cure diseases that threaten life extension. In fact, utopian objectives often appear to increase the average lifespan up to one hundred years of age, as if it were a common objective of the species. At this stage, it is worth asking if it is biologically advisable to attain such an *achievement*. Perhaps it is so outside nature's perspective that it seems like an arrogant audacity, almost as if human beings could not be satisfied with living a few decades and leave room in the planet for the proliferation of life in all its forms and manifestations.

This idea may seem revolutionary or extreme but it must be raised:

> What need is there for the human species to want to prolong its lifespan for so long?

Would it not be another way of disguising the desire of those who dream with a kind of immortality for the privileged few who control the world?

This book tries to demonstrate that the proper word for the beginning of middle age (a long period of years) is not the non-specific *midlife crisis* (only one among a lot of possible psychic symptomatic vicissitudes), but maturescence, when the true beginning of aging can be posed from the actual experience of individuals. Thus, maturescence is defined as the psychic answer to somatic stimuli related to climacterics in men and women.

Chapter 2

Psychoanalysis of maturescence
The onset of middle age and beyond

Introduction (starting from Freud)

This chapter aims at understanding the metapsychology of maturescence based entirely on Freud's texts. This inferred and built theory seeks to delve into an exegesis of maturescence that will put aside some common standpoints which consider that the development of the adult stages of the human vital cycle started and were possible thanks to post-Freudian authors. This could be so in some cases—even though the following text hopes to make evident that Freudian metapsychology also anticipates the possibility of comprehending the issue—because as psychoanalysts, it is essential that we share common Freudian language in order to theorize and debate. Henceforth we hope that each author will start, continue and examine his personal development and not the other way around: making Freud the starting point rather than returning to Freud.

For this reason, each Freudian paragraph has not only been quoted directly but also follows the specific chronological nomenclature established by James Strachey in the British Standard Edition, as well as the corresponding page number, all accompanied by a series of questions regarding the text. Moreover, this author has taken care of differentiating between *instinct* [Instinkt] and *drive* [Trieb], absent in Strachey's translation, which has been extended as a rule and which also makes theoretical interchanges easier. Furthermore, the text also serves as companion to the diagrams included in this edition, which summarize in images the theoretical Freudian path suggested by this author in order to understand maturescence.

This chapter also aims to be a manual for the reader, who may add or remove its contents according to his own psychoanalytical experience, until a personal concept of the proposed theory is elaborated because a metapsychology is essential, regardless of the issue involved: a psychoanalytic clinical interpretation is impossible without a metapsychological base that sustains it.

The author suggests the reader follow the reading of this chapter with the help of Figures 2.1 and 2.2.

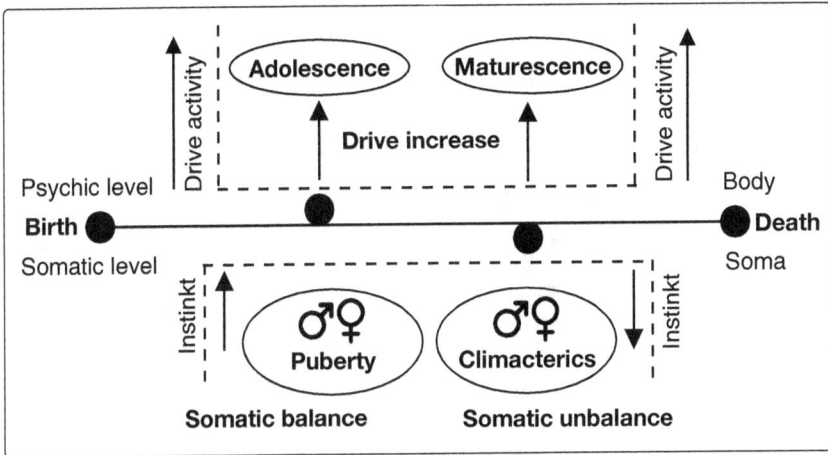

Figure 2.1 Adolescence and maturescence during life cycle.

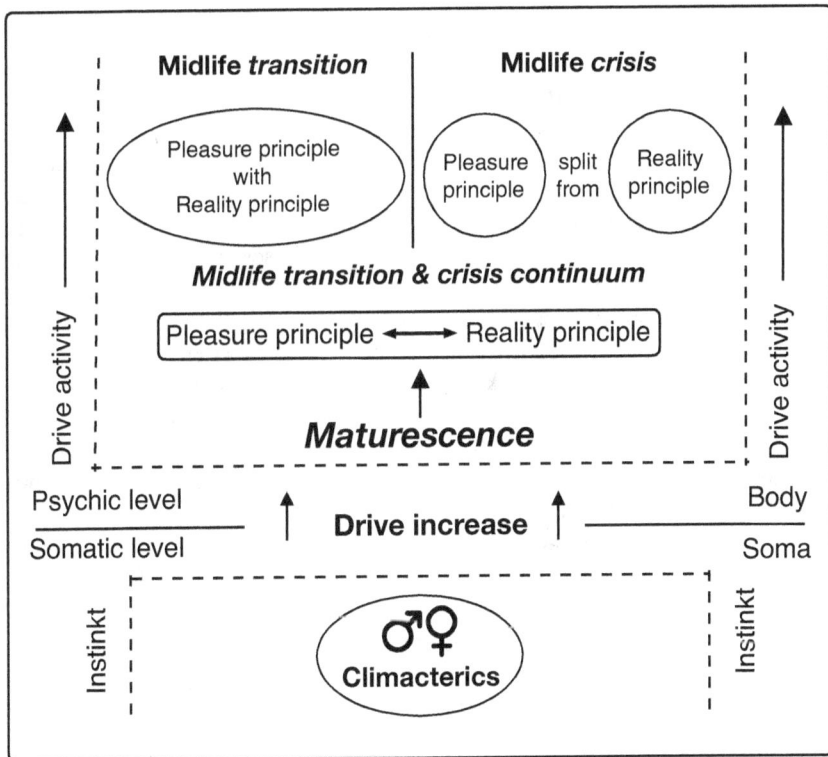

Figure 2.2 Metapsychology of maturescence.

Guide to key Freudian concepts used in the metapsychology of maturescence

- The two main imperatives of the human species.
- Psychoanalysis as a natural science.
- Difference between *Instinkt* (instinct) and *Trieb* (drive).
- Drive increase during climacterics.
- Sleeping and not sleeping dogs.
- The two principles of mental functioning.
- Experience of satisfaction.
- On transience.
- Ego's immortality challenged by reality.
- The Freudian concept of death.
- The painful riddle of death.

Maturescence: the onset of middle age and beyond

There is a specific point at the start of middle age that may be considered as the true beginning of aging: maturescence. Of course, it might be possible to consider the two intermingled sources and paths of aging: somatic aging and psychic aging. The focus of this book tries to demonstrate that aging—true aging—*happens* and *is experienced* from middle age onwards—two different verbs implying different sources and outcomes.

The idea—and clinical evidence confirms this—is that aging *happens* due to an impersonal source, surely related to the uncanny aspects of somatic life; and when this author says that aging *is experienced* from a specific point in the life cycle onwards, he is referring to a psychic source related, in turn, to available personal working-through inner resources. Both sides—the impersonal and the personal—are at work simultaneously when (true) aging begins. There is a tension between what happens and what is experienced, the outcome of which—within this framework—is the phenomenon of human aging.

From a somatic source's perspective, the specific starting point for aging is related to stimuli springing from reproductive functioning loss (women) or decrease (men) (in this case what *happens*). This starting point evinces important somatic landmarks linked to menopause in women and climacterics in men. These important somatic landmarks generate stimuli that require and promote the amount of psychic working-through each individual needs to manage in order to make possible his/her ongoing process of psychic development (what is *experienced*). Thus, the psychological counterpart and outcome, and the proper individual *translation* of these stimuli coming from somatic sources are what we have called maturescence (Montero, 2015), which is mainly related to the body (soma invested with libido and aggression).

Maturescence is the proper word for this psychic process because it is a term that evinces an urge towards growth just as the term *adolescence* does.

The latter derives from the Latin *adolescens–ntis* (3rd conjugation) and means "the one who is growing." It consists of the prefix *ad*: "towards," and the verb *alescere*: "to grow" or "develop." Adolescence means transformation towards adulthood. Maturescence, in turn, means "the one who is becoming mature," or transformation towards maturity, also encompassing the idea of a transformational process.

Maturescence is a prior stage to what psychoanalytic literature has traditionally referred to as *senescence*. A maturescent individual is considered one who has aged but is not yet old. Moreover, it is a truly important moment in the life cycle because it is a stage that encompasses the opportunity human beings have for the renewal of their own subjectivity as well as the development of many other psychic features. The scope of this transcendent psychic working-through urge that occurs around the peri-climacteric period in women and men is evident throughout what was known as midlife crisis, although this book tries to demonstrate the need of a deeper and distinctive way of understanding this psychic process.

The metapsychological exegesis of *maturescence* entails the inextricable link between biological and psychological processes, expressed through drive activity. It is a process that has this starting point and can take many different individual pathways that account for this transformation.

Instinct and its vicissitudes: the (human) *invention* of aging

Reproductive functioning is important for the subject of maturescence. This tenet is based on Freud (1914c) [p. 78] (1915c) [p. 125] (1916–1917 [1915–(1917]) [p. 316] (1920g) [p. 45] (1933a; [1932]) [p. 95] when he considers that the human species comes to life to satisfy two main imperatives.

> The individual does actually carry on a twofold existence: one to serve his own purposes and the other as a link in a chain, which he serves against his will, or at least involuntarily. The individual himself regards sexuality as one of his own ends; whereas from another point of view he is an appendage to his germ-plasm, at whose disposal he puts his energies in return for a bonus of pleasure. He is the mortal vehicle of a (possibly) immortal substance—like the inheritor of an entailed property, who is only the temporary holder of a state which survives him.
>
> (1914c) [p. 78]

The first imperative implies achieving self-satisfaction—the part of the affirmation that poses "to serve his own purposes"—what allows humans a narcissistic acknowledgement through the bond with the self and with external objects as well as the exchange with other generations. This first principle diachronically encompasses the entire individual life cycle. But humans also come to life with another imperative: to reproduce themselves—the part of the affirmation that poses "a link in a chain"—This second principle affects synchronically a particular period: that which takes place once the individual can procreate and ends once he stops being a link in the chain of genetic transmission.

By way of example, we quote another reference from Freud regarding this topic in order to illustrate the importance of August Weismann's thought in Freud's work, a kind of *mentor* on the subject:

> It was he (Weismann) who introduced the division of living substance into mortal and immortal parts. The mortal part is the body in the narrower sense—the soma—which alone is subject to natural death. The germ-cells, on the other hand, are potentially immortal, in so far as they are able, under certain favourable conditions, to develop into a new individual, or, in other words, to surround themselves with a new soma.
>
> (1920g), [p. 45]

Freud (1920g) takes into account Weismann's principles; the latter considered that human beings were the carriers of an immortal substance, a concept he had posed at the turn of the 19th century as the germ-plasm. This concept was reborn in the seventies with Richard Dawkins's (1976) theory of the selfish gene. These concepts have also been dealt with in *The August Weismann legacy*, in the chapter *Background* dealing with theoretical developments about midlife. If an individual somehow succeeds in transmitting the germ-plasm, he/she assures the continuity of life. Thus, reproduction becomes a kind of warranty of a symbolic immortality.

Although these two imperatives are of transcendental importance, the second one must be taken especially into account for the conceptualization of maturescence and subsequent middle age:

> What happens when we are no more necessary for the aim and mandate of the species?
>
> What happens when nature does not need us anymore and we begin our long lasting effort for survival, trying to permanently reach later stages of life?

This author would like to consider that the true *mandate* of the human species is really different from that of individuals because the *mandate* of the human species demands dying after individuals are useless for reproductive purposes, whereas, instead of dying, human beings have *invented* aging, as will be explained below.

The tension between the soma and the body

If human beings are no longer necessary for the species after their climacterics, it is possible to think of the importance that biological reproduction has—considering in this case not only climacterics but also puberty—the two end-moments in the human life cycle where reproduction strives to express itself. We therefore pose three questions:

Why are puberty and climacterics the two most important phases in the heroic myth cycle?

Why are these two important phases as important as birth and death?

Why has humanity needed to express these two phases in its myths?

This author thinks that these two stages are important because exogamy coincides with puberty and the heroic myth cycle's "Descent into Hell" coincides with male and female climacterics. As a result, the hero's somatic processes—physiological, metabolic, hormonal—demand an additional measure of extreme psychic work. The somatic magnitude of these processes could be what has caused civilizations to represent pubescent and climacteric revolutions as phases in the hero's mythical cycle—understanding the hero as an allegory of the immortal double, conveyed in this case as a collective fantasy, as it is expressed in Chapter 7.

Blos (1979) maintains that puberty is an event of nature and adolescence is a human event. Even though the concept *human event* might seem to exclude *humans* from nature, we can discern what Blos is driving at. It may be helpful to stress that, in the context in which Blos made this affirmation, it would have been clearer to postulate that puberty is mainly a biological event and that adolescence is predominantly a psychological consequence of puberty. In both cases, we have a sort of extended biology similar to what Freud proposed concerning the continuum between biology and psychology. Owing to this continuum, Freud always considered psychoanalysis to be a natural science:

Psychoanalysis is a part of the mental science of psychology. Psychology too, is a natural science.

(1940b [1938]) [p. 282]

Moreover:

Each individual somehow recapitulated in an abbreviated form the entire development of the human race.

(1916–1917 [1915–1917]) [p. 199]

From this vertex—psychoanalysis within the natural sciences —we could think of puberty as a phylogenetic landmark and adolescence as its ontogenetic outcome.

Then, just as Blos (1979) points out that initiation into adolescence coincides with measurable somatic milestones (puberty), we can acknowledge that maturescence also coincides with measurable somatic milestones (climacterics) that give birth to specific psychic processes; in the latter case, maturescence itself.

This affirmation may be extended by maintaining that climacterics is mainly biological and maturescence is its psychological outcome, or that climacterics is primarily related to phylogeny and maturescence to ontogeny. From this perspective, we could consider that climacterics occur in the soma—anatomy—and maturescence in the body—the body as the soma invested with libido and aggression, as was already stated. Thus, we could tentatively define maturescence as the result of the tension between the soma and the body, as Ciancio (2014) has already suggested.

This difference is of such importance as to become one of the centers of this way of theorization on maturescence. If soma implies anatomy and body implies psychology, we could find a difference equivalent to the one between instinct and drive, as will be discussed further on.

Equivalently, we could think of a metaphor between need and wish, where *need* may be the source for the somatic expression and *wish* the source for bodily expression. In this case, couldn't it be thought of that need is the necessary counterpart of wish and wish the necessary counterpart of need? Could we think of one without the other?

The relationship, bond and tension between the soma and the body—and its difference—is nuclear in order to understand maturescence. To comprehend the difference between soma and body we would like to bring up the important current concepts of contemporary literary criticism—posed here as a metaphor—which detach *faction* from *fiction*. Faction (from *fact*: something that actually exists; reality; truth) and fiction (from fiction: the art of feigning, inventing, or imagining). The *faction* concept—psychoanalytically near to the concept of *actual*—has a fixed density that brings it closer to the concept of *soma*; whereas the *fiction* concept flows freely just as the *body* can express itself through drive activity.

The revolution produced in the soma—at the metabolic, physiological and hormonal level—is so significant in these two stages of life that it leads to a subjective unbalancing which can drift toward an extreme response as the consequence of the psychic work it brings about. Thus, just as adolescents can be depicted in front of a mirror scrutinizing the *explosion* of their bodies, we can picture maturescent individuals also in front of a mirror bearing witness to their physical *implosion*. Both cases entail uncertainty and fear of some uncanny arousal and, in the case of maturescence, a conscious fear of old age and death.

The two moratoriums [and the (human) *invention* of aging]

But if puberty and climacterics are periods or processes typical of the human life cycle, if they have happened to all human beings since time immemorial, why do they create such an important demand for psychic work? Should we not suppose that what makes us human beings should be experienced as something "natural" instead of something that produces such a tremendous psychic upheaval?

The psychic aspect of extended biology needs to be accommodated because human beings seem to be conditioned by two great moratoriums. The first one is what Erikson (1951) termed the adolescent moratorium and the second could be termed the maturescent moratorium. These (originally anti-natural?) human moratoriums create specific psychic phenomena, both for adolescence and maturescence.

In contemporary western society, the adolescent moratorium requires putting off procreation, even though the biological imperative might peremptorily demand it. The frustration of this post-pubertal demand is what brings on the aforementioned psychic work the thrust towards adolescence as a psychic phenomenon.

Something similar must happen during climacteric stages because they begin a moratorium that puts off another biological imperative; in this case, death. Maturescents are no longer useful for nature's *plan* because they cannot go on procreating, but they resist death by *inventing* old age—a rare phenomenon among other species. The post-climacteric moratorium that puts off dying is a consequence of the instinctive imbalance that characterizes climacterics and accounts for the specific psychic work typical of maturescence.

At this point we should clarify another fact of human nature related to moratoriums. Both adolescent and maturescent moratoriums do not just delay the species' imperatives. Being human is not simply a matter of procreating and dying. During the adolescent moratorium, the individual has sexual intercourse without procreating, whereas in the maturescent moratorium, instead of resigning themselves to death, individuals try to extend their life as long as possible, to go on having sex just for pleasure even though nature's imperative no longer asks them to procreate. This is the reason why, at this stage, both moratoriums experience a feeling of chronic uncertainty and paradox, a psychic characteristic of adolescence and maturescence.

Here it's important to highlight the well-known astonishing popular intuition that midlife (middle age in this author's way of thinking) may be understood as a second adolescence—as depicted also through comics, soap operas, novels and so on. It's as if this intuition were we can fund the psychic confirmation both moratoriums' reality in lay language instead in a psychoanalytic perspective.

Indeed, the enormous demands of sexuality and death for psychic work—in the first and second moratoriums respectively—led to the discovery of psychoanalysis. The importance of this subject, confirmed by the nuclear psychoanalytic postulates, is not only found in the hero's mythical cycle but also in linguistic euphemisms. In fact, euphemisms are alternate expressions or lexical deformations often related to sexuality and death, the core aspects of these moratoriums. This should be of no surprise to psychoanalysts, but it still remains obvious when one examines a specific dictionary of euphemisms

(Rawson, 1995) or seeks direct confirmation in everyday speech. The reader will find further references on this subject in Chapter 6.

Paradoxically, these two postulated moratoriums are points in the life cycle in which true growth and important subjective changes may be achieved—including intersubjective and inter-personal authenticity. For this reason, we can think of maturescence as an opportunity the life cycle provides the individual to promote, continue and deepen his personal development within his own subjectivity (intra-subjectivity) in his relationship with objects (inter-subjectivity) as well as with different generations (trans-subjectivity). Of course, this is what happens in the best situations because psychopathology will always work to exacerbate and make these processes visible, something that in normal development is kept under wraps.

It behooves us to clarify an issue that is a challenge as far as this author is concerned: the male climacteric is very different from the abrupt ending occasioned by menopause of the female climacteric. Even though it is true that the onset of male climacteric does not put an end to procreative activity until the man has entered old age, ethological studies of natural biology have specifically shown that in higher animals—including humans—the offspring of older fathers can be born with physical deformities or with handicaps affecting their survival. It appears that human beings want to deny the similarities of male and female climacterics because their manifestations are so different, even though they are functional equivalents of one another.

In terms of psychoanalytic practice, it is not surprising that both female and male climacterics should have different destinies. The natural violence of female menopause would seem to leave less possibilities of denying the reality of the boundaries of procreation and all the psychic consequences stemming from it. In the case of male climacterics, it is easier to maintain a position of denial, with the equivalent psychic consequences often found as symptomatic during maturescence.

Drives and their vicissitudes

As has already been stated, it is evident that the human species makes an enormous effort to live longer. This phenomenon is one of the founding pillars of psychoanalysis because at one stage of evolution, when instinctive, automatic and repetitive biological life for millions of years had been the same as for the rest of the animal species, psychic life appeared and began to be represented. Aging—as the effort to live longer—emerged with psychic life. What we name *drive* in psychoanalysis is based on that representation of instincts, a concept different from *instinct* itself. That representation also serves as a basis for the enormous difference between the so called animal species and the human species.

Drives are considered an exclusively human attribute. The classic definition of drive is:

An "instinct" [drive] appears to us as a concept on the frontier between the mental and the somatic, as the psychical representative of the stimuli originating from within the organism and reaching the mind, as a measure of the demand made upon the mind for work in consequence of its connection with the body.

(1915c) [p. 120]

Strachey's translation does not yet distinguish between instinct and drive, specified many years later, as has been already stated. Nevertheless, it still is the official definition that led post-Freudian authors to suggest further nuances.

We will now share an amusing story that will allow us to decenter the human perspective in order to understand the transcendental difference between *instinct* and *drive*. It will also serve to understand the *uses* of sexuality, consistent with the second moratorium suggested previously, thus trying to approximate it to a so called *animal* perspective; a positioning undoubtedly difficult for human beings. The provenance of the story that follows will be revealed later:

If your dog had your brain and could speak, and if you asked it what it thought of your sex life, you might be surprised by its response; it would be something like this: Those disgusting humans have sex any day of the month! Barbara proposes sex even when she knows perfectly well that she isn't fertile—like just after her period. John is eager for sex all the time, without caring whether his efforts could result in a baby or not. But if you want to hear something really gross—Barbara and John kept on having sex while she was pregnant! That's as bad as all the times when John's parents come for a visit, and I can hear them too having sex, although John's mother went through this thing they call menopause years ago. Now she can't have babies anymore, but she still wants sex, and John's father obliges her. What a waste of effort! Here's the weirdest thing of all: Barbara and John, and John's parents, close the bedroom door and have sex in private, instead of doing it in front of their friends like any self-respecting dog.

[p. 1]

This amusing story appears at the beginning of *Why Is Sex Fun?* (1997) by the physiologist and evolutionary biologist Jared Diamond. The author considers that it serves as an example in order to change the human-based perspective of what constitutes normal sexual behavior, thus reaching his concept of speciesism, or the self-referred (narcissistic?) style human beings adopted to understand their sexual conduct. He has suggested, therefore, that human sexual conduct is abnormal when compared to most species. As a result, Diamond proposed that a *great leap forward* took place which led to the take-off and definite separation of human beings from the rest of the species. From that moment onwards, humanity began its so called *independence* from the rest of the species.

From the psychoanalytical perspective, however, it would seem that Diamond couldn't think of the issue of *independence* based on the concept of drive. The latter idea would facilitate his thought—but he is not a psychoanalyst—perhaps allowing him to find another way of considering the human species.

Nevertheless, the metaphorical value of Diamond's story serves to illustrate and understand the concept of drive: the behavior of both couples in the story provide a good example of the life drive, unconcerned with procreation—another human invention. That is why the soma (which belongs to instinctive life) becomes the body (which belongs to the life drive).

These concepts about the species' *mandate* lead us to distinguish between the soma and the body. Soma is what gives stimuli whereas body is human soma invested with its own life drive. The soma happens, the body is experienced—as was stated above. The human species has a body because it can represent instinctual life. When instinctual representation became possible, the most important human achievements began as well as the worst disasters, another difference with the rest of the species.

Drive increase and maturescence

This author suggests that true aging begins with the psychic manifestations of peri-climacterics in men and women. These ideas are based on Freud's (1910c) [p. 133] (1912c) [p. 235] (1916–1917 [1915–1917]) [p. 402] (1937c) [p. 226] because on several occasions he writes that around menopause, and often at the age of fifty in men, there is a drive increase that fosters a neurotic mental state (maturescence?).

In his essay *Leonardo da Vinci and a Memory of his Childhood*, Freud refers for the first time to drive increase in men around fifty:

> At the summit of his life, when he was in his early fifties—a time when in women the sexual characters have already undergone involution and when in men the libido not infrequently makes a further energetic advance.
>
> (1910c) [p. 133]

Here we find the more empirical Freud. At that time no one had acknowledged what we today identify as the male climacteric nor its drive related impressions, but Freud came upon its effects in his clinical work, which is why he was able to attribute this "energetic advance" to men.

The next time Freud refers to drive increase beyond puberty is in *Types of Onset of Neurosis*, on this occasion with a whole metapsychological explanation:

We see people fall ill who have hitherto been healthy, who have met with no fresh experience and whose relation to the external world has undergone no change, so that the onset of their illness inevitably gives an impression of spontaneity. A closer consideration of such cases, however, shows us that none the less a change has taken place in them whose importance we must rate very highly as a cause of illness. As a result of their having reached a particular period of life, and in conformity with regular biological processes, the *quantity* [italics in the original] of libido in their mental economy has experienced an increase which is in itself enough to upset the equilibrium of their health and to set up the necessary conditions for a neurosis. It is well known that more or less sudden increases of libido of this kind are habitually associated with puberty and the menopause—with the attainment of a certain age in women; in some people they may in addition be manifested in periodicities that are still unknown.

(1912c) [p. 235]

This last paragraph is essential because it contains a complete foundation for the metapsychology of maturescence. It alludes to the apparent spontaneity of illness; it correlates synchronic "biological processes" with a particular "period of life"; it indicates how libidinal increase upsets the healthy equilibrium to foster neurosis and it explicitly addresses puberty and menopause.

We will not continue with the series of alluded references; the reader can resort to them, since the names of the papers and page numbers have been provided. However, we could point out that possibly Freud was unable to directly link this drive increase with the somatic instinctual source because at that moment the work of hormonal activity was not so clear, although it had already been discovered. True research in this area began a bit later than Freud's statements, but the ideas for a theory of maturescence seem to be already there.

A drive increase during adolescence, due to hormonal upsurge, is easier to conceive, but how would it be possible to think of an equivalent drive increase around male and female climacterics, if hormonal activity is decreasing? This author believes that Freud's great intuition has to do with the outcome of somatic unbalance; in this case we could refer to hormonal unbalance, if we want to detach a single variable. Unbalance always demands an extreme urge of psychic work: "a measure of the demand made upon the mind for work in consequence of its connection with the body" (Freud, 1915c) [p. 120], as previously quoted. This occurs because instinct is a different concept from drive: instinct may increase or decrease, but the representation of this somatic activity has a psychic resonance that may be psychoanalytically understood as drive—and drives, once they are set in motion, always demand psychic work.

Once drives are set in motion to promote psychic work, they must be taken into account—it is interesting to highlight the actual factor for this theorization—as can be seen from the following citation that complements the previous series:

If an instinctual conflict is not a present one and does not manifest itself in any way, it cannot be influenced by analysis. The warning that we should "let sleeping dogs lie"—as we are so often told in connection with our investigation of the psychic underworld—is peculiarly inapposite when applied to the relations existing in psychic life. For, if the instincts are causing disturbances it is a proof that the dogs are not sleeping and if it is evident that they really are sleeping, we have not the power to wake them.

(1937c) [p. 386]

Here lies the transcendence of the *actual* factor, since nothing can be done if the dogs are quiet and not barking. It could be thought that in order to get the maturescent process going, we would need to awaken the dogs and set them in motion. This, however, goes beyond the active search of a psychoanalyst because it would depend on somatic factors. In other words, the processing characteristic of maturescence can only be activated from the somatic source. If the drive activity does not barge in, it is because the somatic imbalance demanded by psychic work has not yet been set in motion: "a measure of the demand made upon the mind for work in consequence of its connection with the body" (1915c) [p. 120], again, to continue with the definition of drive used previously.

This astonishing Freudian intuition—drive increase during climacterics—is what allows this author to make an essentially Freudian conceptualization of maturescence, forthcoming middle age and aging. From that moment on, after universal somatic climacterics and forthcoming psychical drive increase, different vicissitudes present themselves for each individual. Each person will work-through with his own inner resources—complementary series, ego defensive mechanisms, ideal ego or ego ideal preponderancy, availability for mourning processes, split or repression's psychic organization, narcissistic or object tendency, etc.—this urge of an extra psychic work that Freud named drive increase.

From this vertex we make Edmund Bergler's (1954) words our own. Bergler defined midlife—in his case using the concept of middle-age—long before Jaques (1965) did, as a *revolt against biology*, a fight against the biological mandate that shows the extreme urge of psychic work, termed maturescence in this book. When the *revolt against biology* happens, the individual experiences the need to do something. This author poses it as a universal because it is a measure of psychic work that may be externally noticeable in those individuals with fewer resources for an authentic working-through process. Furthermore, it will be less externally noticeable in individuals who simply try to renew their lives taking advantage of the different vicissitudes this drive increase may foster towards new creative, positive and developmental paths.

Perhaps a clinical example taken from Freud (1933a [1932]) could be proposed in order to pose the question:

Why does the internal change that takes place during the second half of life that Freud proposes take place?

Could we consider once again the drive increase factor acting in the patient, as was alluded to by Freud?

So it may easily happen that the second half of a woman's life may be filled by the struggle against her husband, just as the shorter first half was filled by her rebellion against her mother. When this reaction has been lived through, a second marriage may easily turn out very much more satisfying.

[p. 133]

Again, following Freud, psychopathology shows macroscopically what development shows microscopically, but both core psychic processes are the same, regardless of how we name them. Somehow we could refer to a maturescent crisis and a maturescent transition, for example, as being both ends of a continuum—mostly acting-out defensive mechanisms and depressive defensive mechanisms at work in the first case; and mostly mourning processes at work in the second, regardless of the consideration that each individual psychic working-through process is unique.

Pleasure principle and reality principle: the search for satisfaction

The following introductory explanation proposes a metapsychology of drive increase due to climacterics unbalance in men and women and opens up the possibility for further research on the subject. If we are to understand and be able to provide an interpretation of maturescence, psychoanalysis must understand psychic content within the framework of metapsychology. It is time, therefore, for a tentative definition of maturescence.

Maturescence is defined as the psychic outcome related to the true beginning of biological aging. It is fostered, featured and shaped through a universal drive increase, which Freud (1910c) [p. 133] (1912c) [p. 235] (1916–1917 [1915–1917]) [p. 402] (1937c) [p. 226] already linked to climacteric phenomena in men and women. Each individual will work-through these tensions with his own psychic resources, allowing the manifestation of a series of personal paths depicting different subjective landscapes. But the measure of psychic work activated by this drive increase could promote a renewed *experience of dissatisfaction* that becomes evident through the psychic processing required. However, we should not confuse the *experience of dissatisfaction* with Freud's proposition of experience of an external fright (1900a):

Let us examine the antithesis to the primary experience of satisfaction—namely, the experience of an external fright.

[p. 600]

This experience of dissatisfaction is mainly useful for the understanding of maturescent response to drive increase.

Why does this *experience of dissatisfaction* occur?
What could be understood as *experience of dissatisfaction* if psychoanalysis precisely defines the experience of satisfaction as the setting in motion of psychic life and wish fulfillment?

Please note the highlighted idea that the goal of human experience is the *search for satisfaction* and not the mere *search for pleasure*.
In this regard, Freud (1926e) argues:

> We assume that the forces which drive the mental apparatus into activity are produced in the bodily organs as an expression of the major somatic needs. We give these bodily needs, in so far as they represent an instigation to mental activity, the name of "*Trieb*" [drive]. What, then, do these instincts [drive] want? Satisfaction—that is, the establishment of situations in which the bodily needs can be extinguished.
>
> [p. 200]

The *search for pleasure* ends up implying a simple process that tends towards the zero discharge, emptying the psychic landscape; whereas the *search for satisfaction* implies a more complex kind of processing that includes several other factors: the object, the specific somatic action, etc., following the Freudian model of the experience of satisfaction (1950a [1887–1902]) [p. 317ff] (1900a) [p. 565].

The experience of satisfaction involves the simultaneous fulfillment (coincidence) of the pleasure principle (primary process) and the reality principle (secondary process), as can be inferred in Freud's *Project for a Scientific Psychology* (1950a [1887–1902]) [p. 317ff] and *The Interpretation of Dreams* (1900a) [p. 565]. Consequently, the renovated tension and its eventual dissociation (splitting) between both principles will be the cause of the *experience of dissatisfaction*.

Even though from an evolutionary perspective the relay of the pleasure principle by the reality principle is to be expected, this process is permanently reversible—for example, in the daily experience of dreams. It is for this reason that Freud (1911b) explains:

> The supersession of the pleasure principle by the reality principle, with all the psychical consequences involved, is not in fact accomplished all at once; nor does it take place simultaneously all along the line.
>
> [p. 222]

Likewise, Freud (1916–1917 [1915–1917]) highlights the value of both principles for the ego's development, always considering the usefulness of the reversibility of both principles of mental functioning.

The transition from the pleasure principle to the reality principle is one of the most important steps forward in the ego's development.

[p. 357]

This last observation helps us to understand the violence of the maturescent drive increase, which is one of the most common factors that intensify the tension between the reality principle and the pleasure principle, promoting and fostering the experience of dissatisfaction through its tendency towards splitting. This is the cause of the so called midlife crisis.

Of course, drive increase not only depends on the climacteric somatic imbalance but it is also influenced by constitutional factors and the predominant psychopathology. These factors push against the natural tension and bond between pleasure principle and reality principle promoting the *experience of dissatisfaction*.

There are two main extreme paths for this psychic situation. The first path implies the prevalence of the extreme of reality dissociated from the extreme of pleasure. It may lead to a subjection experienced as lives without content, hollow, anonymous, meaningless, almost like a phenomenon of empty depression. Individuals often refer to this state as surrendering to the *routine of everyday life*, as if no further chances existed to renew their lives.

The second path implies the prevalence of the extreme of pleasure dissociated from the extreme of reality, leading to a kind of psychic functioning where the ideal ego with its demand of *immortality* and the immediate discharge into action predominates; where the balance between the ideal ego and the ego ideal is also lost. Individuals often refer to this state as a new opportunity to recover past times, thinking they will achieve an ultimate renewal that guarantees them eternal youth.

Both extremes condemn subjectivity to dead-end situations despite being ego-syntonic for the individual—although specific drive increase is experienced as ego-dystonic and fosters psychic working-through. In addition, these extremes could be the result of a splitting factor which the demand of psychic work promotes through the maturescent drive increase. Here the clinical example taken from Freud (1933a [1932]) [p. 133] gains importance once again.

In line with this proposal, it is simple to apply the parallel between both principles to the ego, since the ego has an aspect associated with pleasure (primary process) and another one associated with reality (secondary process), not only in its epigenesis but also in its definitive functioning.

Here it becomes essential to contemplate a vicissitude that is clinically very frequent. Many maturescent patients maintain in their psychoanalytical treatments that they do not have time to do all that they wish, either because they have lost many years neurotically or because they do not have many years to live. Both reasonings imply the resistance to understand precisely the transformational power of wish—especially during maturescent drive increase—

since wish truly opens psychic reality to space and time. A broadening of psychic space is needed for the challenge of a continuing growth, whereas the subjective perception of time, can also be expanded when wish is taken into account. From this perspective, then, maturescent drive increase not only implies the risk that the tension between reality and pleasure be dissociated—as previously sustained—but rather that the irruption of wish through drive increase can promote destinies as surprising as this psychic broadening of space and time in order to achieve authentic satisfaction.

Maturescent transition and maturescent crisis

If the importance of somatic unbalance related to the difficulty and loss of reproductive functioning in maturescence is taken into account, then it would also be useful to consider *On Transience* as a framework for these ideas. In this paper, Freud (1916a [1915]) identifies three possible dispositions that can arise in the face of the transitory (perishing), that is, in what is fated to disappear. These dispositions are closely related to the possibility, the difficulty or the impossibility of psychic re-signification during maturescence. These dispositions are three transformations depicting different pathways.

The first modality implies a series of continuous working-through microprocesses that lead to a new equilibrium:

Transience value is scarcity in time.

[p. 305]

This first attitude concerning the transient nature of existence implies the activation of mourning processes that enables psychic change and assigns (an always relative process of) re-signification to maturescence.

The second modality is a slowing down (stagnation):

An aching despondency.

[p. 305]

This attitude towards the transient nature of existence implies a gradual detaining and consequent chronification of certain personal stereotypes that eventually encompass self-esteem. This could result in an inability to initiate new plans or projects, as if time had stopped. This second modality entails a psychopathological and melancholic way of dealing with transience, making psychic change and re-signification difficult, which, could lead, in turn, to a precarious maturescent working-through.

The third modality is acceleration (an apparent external change):

The rebellion against the fact asserted.

[p. 305]

This acceleration entails the attempt to flee into the past, vertiginously hoping to *recover* bygone times. In this modality a poorly regulated self-esteem may be found: in these circumstances, people engage in various plans or projects with the sole purpose of recovering their youth in a utopian manner. This third modality entails a manic psychopathological way of handling transience, making psychic change and re-signification more difficult. In a manner similar to the second modality, this situation leads to a precarious maturescent working-through.

Again, these three modalities are the consequence of "a measure of the demand made upon the mind for work in consequence of its connection with the body" (Freud, 1915c) [p. 120]. All of them have only individual working-through processing.

If we now take into account the aforementioned considerations, it is possible to postulate a pathognomonic continuum between maturescent transition (first modality) and maturescent crisis (second and third modalities). There would be a transition pole and a crisis pole at opposite ends of this maturescent continuum. From this perspective, each person would experience both a transition and a crisis simultaneously, although transitions and crises would be of different proportions in each mixture.

The proposed continuum leads to the conclusion that maturescent transition and crisis have an inversely proportional relationship, keeping in mind that, although libido and aggression always work simultaneously, maturescent transition could tend towards the fusion of drives whereas maturescent crisis could tend towards a greater diffusion of drives.

Psychopathology during maturescent transition and crisis

The psychic work that a maturescent transition demands points directly toward the recovery of *Selbstgefühl*, in Freudian terms (1914c), or the notion of self and self-esteem. "Every remnant of the primitive feeling of omnipotence which his experience has confirmed" [p. 98] would be changed at the outset of maturescence because then a narcissistic crisis arises that may have different manifestations. In any case, including when the process can be carried out in continuous working-through micro-processes of re-signification, what assumes center stage is a certain functioning of the self. This can be understood as a self-esteem regulator, since the acknowledgement of one's own finite nature implies narcissistic wounds that often initiate the experience of pain, abandonment and personal devaluation.

In the continuous working-through micro-processes (re-signification), the ego evinces a preponderant type of ego-reality work. However, while the content of fantasies often connotes tolerance of what is becoming transient, imperfect or perishing, fantasies generally express an integration between what someone has accomplished and what has not come to pass—especially in the terrain of the ego ideal. From a psychopathological viewpoint, this sort of psychic operation could correspond to psycho-neurosis; and from the perspective of the self, to a cohesive functioning and an adequate regulation of self-esteem.

In melancholic processing (slowing-down, stagnation) and in manic processing (external acceleration, apparent change), there are two different ways of working-through. In both ways the ego's preponderant functional modality corresponds to the ego's archaic functioning (ego-initial reality and ego-pleasure). In the slowing down (stagnation) processing, the preponderant fantasy expresses a total loss, a feeling that the individual can expect nothing from life, whereas in the acceleration process there is an apparent change—fantasies expressing a Proustian attempt to recover times gone by. Both *solutions* imply psychopathology because they are related to narcissistic pathologies, especially to the limitations that the functioning of ego-pleasure imposes. This can be found, fundamentally, in borderline disorders. From the perspective of the self, melancholic processing is related to narcissistic personality disorders and manic processing is linked to narcissistic behavior disorders.

These attempts at recovering self-esteem can also be understood, following Freud (1924e), from auto-plastic and allo-plastic perspectives [p. 185]. In melancholic processing, auto-plastic modifications could be found when experiencing the characteristic loss of worth as well as a generalized sense of meaninglessness (a modification of the internal environment), giving rise to a kind of delusion of inferiority, as suggested by Freud (1917e [1915]) in *Mourning and Melancholia* [p. 246]. On the other hand, in manic processing, symptomatic allo-plastic modifications could be brought on by attempts to recover self-esteem through evident changes in manifest behavior (modification of the external environment). These latter vicissitudes entail narcissistic denial and idealization mechanisms. The manic processing modality (acceleration, apparent change) corresponds to the so called classic midlife or middle age crises, also known as the Gauguin syndrome or, more colloquially as the *midday demon*.

In a way it could be said that specific psychic goings-on that come about during maturescent working-through—due to drive increase brought on by climacteric unbalance—are also relatively independent from psychopathology. That is, even though they are factors to keep in mind, severe narcissistic psychopathology does not necessarily determine or condition the difficulty or the inability to process the phenomena of maturescence.

At any rate, drive increase adds a vertex to psychopathology that allows a broader and simultaneously deeper understanding of maturescence. In addition, although drive increases are also expressed in clinical material, they should not lead the psychoanalyst to pay them special attention during the session; instead, the analyst should be working in the *absolute present*, as it occurs according to nature's *plan*, which has no particular *human* purposes or acknowledgment of past or future.

Several universals (invariants) in maturescence

Even if the tension between the soma and the body is, par excellence, something that has been deemed, following Freud, "the most touchy point in the narcissistic system, the immortality of the ego, which is so hard pressed by reality" (1914c) [p. 91], it is an empirical constant and the main source of stimuli for the onset of maturescence.

Consequently, it is possible to identify several metapsychological factors in order to understand the particular psychic work that re-signification requires to deal with maturescence. Although these factors are all interconnected, they will be considered separately for didactic purposes. Being psychic invariants, they have the advantage of overcoming the different vicissitudes that each individual may have to deal with. These constants allow us to study their transformations, which necessarily includes individual differences.

In the first place, once the individual experiences his mourning processes, he will be better able to take on the psychic work demanded by maturescence. Evidences of the mourning process's failure can be seen in certain individuals who make their maturescent parental function more adolescent in an attempt to dissolve the natural asymmetry between parent and child.

In a direct line with the above topic, maturescence could also entail updating the ego ideal. As the representative of symbolic ideals, the ego ideal plans for a future state of affairs, as Hanly (1983) states—whenever this future state of affairs can be accepted by the subject, or facts, if the ideal ego representing narcissistic ideals re-emerge. These narcissistic ideals require a state of being, as Hanly also suggests, where the passing of time has been abolished.

These assumptions led this author to pose the idea that between the ideal ego and the ego ideal one would find a relationship equivalent to the one between a hero and a man. Contrary to the ordinary docile ego ideal, which tries to work things through, the individual finds the ideal ego's heroic tyranny, which demands immediate fulfillment of the chronic desires of immortality (Montero, 2015).

Maturescence also implies a reactivation of the pre-Oedipal and Oedipal conflicts.

Freud (1931d), states:

> The Oedipus complex, as far as we know, is present in childhood in all human beings, undergoes great alterations during the years of development and in many individuals is found in varying degrees of strength even at a mature age.
>
> [p. 251]

Actual losses and threats of further losses reactivate the schizoid conflict (abandonment anxiety). With respect to the Oedipal conflict (castration anxiety), maturescence facilitates the re-emergence of parricidal and incestuous fantasies. It is important to mention here that the re-emergence of the Oedipal conflict also occurs in people who may have lost their parents early on or who have never had children. That is, even though one might think that such people were never linked to symbolic parental equivalences, they too would fall prey to the reactions that appear during maturescence.

Finally and naturally, as part of dealing with the maturescent working-through processing, it is important to highlight the revision and re-elaboration of one's primary and secondary identifications. These identifications would be directly related to the ideal ego and the ego ideal. They would suffer the same de-identification vicissitudes and a subsequent new identification and would always be susceptible to revision. As a characteristic process during matures-cence, de-identification entails a distancing from and a relinquishing of one's own parental and social discourse. As an eventual path toward dealing with generational telescoping, as Faimberg (2005) states, it also entails a reconsideration and connection with one's own discourse or idiom, following Bollas's (1989) considerations and differences between fate and destiny.

The tension between the soma and the body and, following Freud (1914c) "the immortality of the ego, which is so hard pressed by reality" [p. 91], added to the elements detailed above, are the metapsychological bases that allow us to infer the sort of psychic work maturescence requires.

What are we referring to when we speak about death?

We have often listened to our patients worried or scared about their own death. Usually, when a patient says any word, we search for its unconscious meaning; however, when the patient mentions the word *death*, this does not happen, and the psychoanalyst takes for granted what the patient is referring to: his death in itself.

From a psychoanalytical point of view, as was already mentioned, matures-cent drive increase hinges on Freud's (1914c):

> The most touchy point in the narcissistic system, the immortality of the ego, which is so hard pressed by reality
>
> [p. 91]

This is what appears as pain in the face of the inevitable: one's own aging and eventual death.

Seen from the logic of a kind of *navel of maturescence*—if we try to find a deeper level of understanding—the perception of one's own aging and death is similar to what happens in Plato's cave (*The Republic*, 7). The cave inhabit-ants can see the shadows projected on the wall but they do not know they are being projected, which is equivalent to what goes on in dream-work, as it was stated in the chapter *Mid-life: Steps to be taken before the introduction of a new concept*. Given this, we can imagine that the aging that concerns maturescent individuals is the aging associated with the second moratorium, something very hard to psychically acknowledge—here the tension between what *happens* and what is *experienced* is again in the forefront.

Two ways of understanding these issues can be suggested at this point. In the first case, the maturescent moratorium is *especially* related to what happens to a person in the present. For this reason, a vertex could be proposed that may be called *the experience with death in the present*, which is the expression of the soma. What happens at this level of maturescence is untenable, inadmissible, incomprehensible and ineffable because it implies the presence of a biological footprint that cannot be represented in the maturescent present; for this reason, the *natural* drive increase demands an extra level of psychic work.

In the second instance, the maturescent moratorium could be called *the experience with death in the future*, which is the expression of the body. This implies a different working-through psychic activity, according to what the individual is able to experience. This is so because future death has *yet to* happen, especially if we keep in mind the definition of trauma entailing events that threaten or overwhelm the representational abilities of the psychic apparatus. We stress the words *yet to* because they indicate an occurrence that *still* and *up to a particular moment* has not happened, but which will inexorably come to pass. And that which is *yet to* happen constitutes a psychic presence that is as good as real, that is always felt in advance and is generally threatening because it pertains to the second moratorium. In this case, maturescents can displace into the future whatever subjective experience they might have at a particular time in the present. The *navel of maturescence* implies the tension between *the experience of death in the present* (soma) and *the experience of death in the future* (body), leading to a kind of uncertainty that can be quite painful.

If we take into account the very frequent and extreme reactions (transformations) that the psychic apparatus needs to employ so as to negotiate maturescence, we can deduce that such an extreme defense must be related to an extreme and unmanageable pain, making it possible to infer the magnitude of psychic work and defenses demanded.

One should also pose the following objection to this point of view:

Why would people worry about death?

The concept of death in Freud's works

Continuing with Freud's (1915b) thought, it seems appropriate to introduce a chronological series of ideas regarding the place and function *death* has in psychic life. In *Thoughts for the Times on War and Death*, he writes:

> It is indeed impossible to imagine our own death; and whenever we attempt to do so we can perceive that we are in fact still present as spectators. Hence

the psycho-analytic school could venture on the assertion that at bottom no one believes in his own death, or, to put the same thing in another way, that in the unconscious every one of us is convinced of his own immortality.

[p. 289]

In the same text, he sustains:

Our habit is to lay stress on the fortuitous causation of the death—accident, disease, infection, advanced age; in this way we betray an effort to reduce death from a necessity to a chance event.

[p. 290]

He also refers to the notion of the unmodified continuity of unconscious nuclear contents, suggesting that death has the same *existence* in the unconscious which primitive man had: none. In *The Uncanny*, Freud (1919h) explains the concept:

There is scarcely any other matter, however, upon which our thoughts and feelings have changed so little since the very earliest times, and in which discarded forms have been so completely preserved under a thin disguise, as our relation to death.

[p. 241]

Our unconscious has as little use now as it ever had for the idea of its own mortality.

[p. 242]

Freud also took it upon himself to explain the human psyche's inability to represent its own death:

Death is an abstract concept with a negative content for which no unconscious correlative can be found

(1923b) [p. 58]

In another paper, Freud (1926d [1925]) also states:

The unconscious seems to contain nothing that could give any content to our concept of the annihilation of life

[p. 123]

Thus, the impossibility of representation reflected in the above citations adds new evidence to the enormous dimension brought about by the second moratorium.

Perhaps the true problem is not death itself. Following Freud (1923b) [p. 58]—as previously stated—we know it would be hardly possible to represent it because the psychic apparatus device makes the representation of personal death impossible. Again, this author wonders what the patient really means every time he utters the word *death*:

Could it be possible that what the patient is referring to has a deeper significance?

But the fact remains that death continues to plunge us into the equivalent abyss experienced by the very first human being, after he could represent his instinctual life through what we psychoanalysts understand as *drive*. We suffer from the same worries that original human being felt—nothing has changed. And we suffer because *death* has no representation and will never have.

Freud (1915b) holds that:

What, we ask, is the attitude of our unconscious towards the problem of death? The answer must be: almost exactly the same as that of primaeval man. In this respect, as in many others, the man of prehistoric times survives unchanged in our unconscious. Our unconscious, then, does not believe in its own death; it behaves as if it were immortal. What we call our "unconscious"—the deepest strata of our minds, made up of instinctual impulses—knows nothing that is negative, and no negation; in it contradictories coincide. For that reason it does not know its own death, for to that we can give only a negative content. Thus there is nothing instinctual in us which responds to a belief in death.

[p. 296]

This is why within this Freudian (1927c) attempt of conceptualization of aging we highlight the Freudian concept of *the painful riddle of death*:

But no one is under the illusion that nature has already been vanquished; and few dare hope that she will ever be entirely subjected to man. There are the elements, which seem to mock at all human control: the earth, which quakes and is torn apart and buries all human life and its works; water, which deluges and drowns everything in a turmoil; storms, which blow everything before them; there are diseases, which we have only recently recognized as attacks by other organisms; and finally there is *the painful riddle of death*, against which no medicine has yet been found, nor probably will be. With these forces nature rises up against us, majestic, cruel and inexorable; she brings to our mind once more our weakness and helplessness, which we thought to escape through the work of civilization.

[p. 16]

With this powerful metaphor, Freud is stating that *the painful riddle of death* has no solution, while simultaneously *the painful riddle of death* is the solution. Everyone is individually free and open in his capacity and psychic condition to make it possible or not to cope with what is activated when we are no more necessary to the so called *plan* of the human species as we begin our aging process.

With this Freudian concept we have the possibility as analysts to be free from the need of attempting an answer to *the painful riddle of death* (Oedipus' riddle of the Sphynx, again?). Conversely, we can simply try to accompany our patients in finding their own paths with respect to this painful riddle; the same is valid with ourselves. Fortunately, this perspective lets us confront this issue with uncertainty and paradox working as the enigmatic components of *the painful riddle of death*.

Why is aging regarded as a problem?

Maturescent individuals wonder about death, particularly their own, in many different ways. However, it is important to psychoanalytically look into the reasons that can lead from the simple conscious question about death to the more *popular* extremes of the midlife crisis: the effort to remain young ("I'll defeat aging and I'll be young forever" or "time doesn't count for me") or depressive or stagnating states of the mind ("everything is lost" or "I have run out of time"), because sometimes the notion of *aging* remains misunderstood. Again:

Why is *aging* regarded as a problem?

One answer may be that this is so when it has become evident that the individual is not developing anymore and has stopped his growth. Otherwise, the passing of time and the different ages in life may be *naturally* lived because aging and death are our *natural* human destinies (emphasis added twice in the word *naturally* and *natural*, following the scope of these ideas).

We have listened to our patients and ourselves many times worried or scared about death, as if this concept were an equivalent concept for aging. This author wonders what we really mean when patients or psychoanalysts say or listen to the word *death*—of course, when there is no somatic pathology or negative prognosis.

We have already mentioned why, when a patient says any word, the psychoanalyst tries to find its most unconscious meaning about what he is trying to convey, but when the patient utters the word *death* it's usually taken for granted that he is speaking about what is called *death*. Perhaps the true problem of aging is not *death* itself. Following Freud (1923b) [p. 58], we know it would be hardly possible to represent death because the psychic apparatus device makes the representation of personal *death* impossible. In this respect, we share Ernest Jones's (1927) concept of *aphanisis*: the fear of the disappearance of sexual desire. It seems that when the patient usually employs the word *death,* he is afraid of the disappearance of his own sexual desire and/or becoming unable of being desired:

What happens if I can't keep on desiring sexually an object?

And from the object vertex:

What if no object desires me anymore?

This logic enables us to interpret what really happens around and especially after maturescence, when what we call maturescence and forthcoming later stages of life begin. *Aphanisis* has always been there, but it suddenly resurfaces during climacteric drive increase—in men and women—as the hidden side, because it tries to find a resolution to a tension that dwells within the individual, leading to a renewed psychic working-through process.

Then, first answer: Aging is regarded as a problem because it conveys the fear of aphanisis—the underlying hidden side of drive increase—the authentic psychic content for aging and death.

But if we follow with the question:

Why is aging regarded as a problem?

Now a tentative answer. Recently this author felt interested and attracted to several truths long taken for granted and tried to find their current validity. There seems to be a kind of *dictatorship of the living matter*—the proposed concept. *Living matter*—human beings in this case—when they live their own lives, suppose, as if it were an illusion, that they *are* defeating death.

This proposed *dictatorship of the living matter* also confirms a nuclear psychoanalytic basis: sex and death. In fact, it is already known that each generation re*discovers* a kind of freedom related to sexual life, in the belief it is obtaining something new. In this regard, Anzieu (1986) writes:

> Every period believes itself to be the first to have discovered sexuality and to have dared to discuss it openly: in this respect, modern society is particularly vain and long-winded.
>
> [p. 89]

It seems that with death the same thing occurs because each period believes they are postponing or defeating death in some way.

Then, the question would be:

Is it true that we contemporaries are *defeating* death?

We consider it appropriate to mention at this stage the research made by Simon Critchley in *The Book of Dead Philosophers* (2009). Although it is centered in the cause of death of more than two hundred philosophers, the ages the majority of them had when they died caught our attention, especially since it belied the fact that in ancient times people supposedly did not live as long as they do now. This author wishes to point out that those who died young did so because they were either murdered or for many other reasons, including suicide. In short, this information is quite surprising, but confirms the reality of the *dictatorship of the living matter*.

Similar findings appear in the investigations of Christine Cave and Oxenham (2017), an Australian anthropologist. She decided to exhume the skeletal remains at early Anglo-Saxon cemeteries. Employing a method used to study the deterioration of dental pieces, she was able to discover the age of the owners of those dental pieces at the time of death. Surprisingly, the majority had had long lives.

We could consider that, as long as we are alive, we are subject to this *dictatorship of the living matter*, which forces us to believe that we are defeating death, postponing it like never before as much as possible; it is a kind of omnipotence of the living matter implying an eternal present that leads the individual to think it is possible to overcome death.

For this reason, the dreams of an eternal youth, of reaching the age of one hundred, of being able to live forever, have passed from one generation to another, as it was done from the beginning of humanity—they were not captured in heroic myths or religious mysticism nor in the intentions of medieval alchemists but have remained alive within humans up to now.

This has led us to question the supposed truth that we are coming close to defeating death or, at least, that we are succeeding in putting it off as much as possible. Perhaps the time has come to consider these (current) *truths* from a humbler perspective, since they may work as false comfort to our narcissism.

Another version of the *dictatorship of the living matter* leads some people to affirm that maturescence occurs nowadays at a later stage of life than before ("Yes, now it's possible," they say). The answer to this assertion is also negative, because nowadays maturescence is simply more visible. However, being processes that constitute us as human beings, they are very ancient and dwell within us from time immemorial despite having become more noticeable due to current cultural and social conditions as a species. Nevertheless, nothing could have changed in terms of the unconscious life of individuals in just fifty or one hundred years of history because it is too short a time. If the evolution of human beings across millions of years is a brief puff, we can imagine how brief that puff would be when referring to fifty or one hundred years ago.

Then, second answer: The problem of aging compels human beings to live with the consolation of the *dictatorship of the living matter*.

Odysseus and the natural position

We would now like to discuss what we have termed *the natural position*, which refers to the acknowledgment of uncertainty and paradox. This is so because uncertainty and paradox are the *natural* consequence of the resolution of the maturescent drive increase.

In order to illustrate what is being proposed, we would like to refer to two literary examples. The first one has to do with the famous poem by Robert

Frost (1874–1963), "The Road not Taken" (1916). The poem's speaker is faced with the dilemma of a road with forking paths, challenging him to make a decision. Which path should he follow? We should highlight here the word *decision*, since it directly aims at the experience of uncertainty and paradox. If we interpret this metaphor as the moments in our lives when we must choose between two or more alternatives—a dilemma which most human beings frequently experience—any choice marks the course of the destiny to be followed. When the poet himself was questioned regarding the poem's ambiguity, he sustained that the actual choice was not really significant, since one would always yearn for the path(s) not taken, reflecting once again the tension leading from the paradox towards the experience of uncertainty.

Between the two paths, the narrator chooses "the one less traveled," giving him the liberty to invest in the renovation of a life project, as suggested by the experience of uncertainty proposed at the beginning of the psychic work characteristic of maturescence.

For the psychoanalyst, what emerges here is the problem of repetitive compulsion, perhaps the other side of the uncertainty experience. When the narrator takes the road less traveled, he challenges repetitive compulsion in order to attempt something different.

The poem's speaker manifests that he knows that the choice taken will affect the rest of his life: nothing can repeat itself, since any choice will have changed everything. One's choices in life, in other words, will always keep the discarded options in the background: uncertainty and paradox in its purest state as the motor of a search. This is precisely what we are attempting to put forward as the path of maturescence towards true maturity.

A similar example appears in the novel *The Sea, The Sea* (1978) by Iris Murdoch (1919–1999), which perhaps alludes to Frost's poem and has a lot to do with the topic of uncertainty. The narrator refers to the inevitable fact that all human beings are presented with choices that can prove beneficial or harmful. With hindsight, of course, the magnitude of previous decisions becomes evident, even though what led us to them has perhaps been forgotten. Such divergent dilemmas, which have inevitably implied foregoing other possibilities, occur in everyone's life.

Finally, we would like to refer to an episode in Homer's *Odyssey* when Odysseus, on his way back home to meet his wife Penelope and his son Telemachus, orders his sailors to tie him to the ship's mast and to put wax in their ears so that he alone may hear the sirens; the latter, however, are not sensual, voluptuous and beautiful women with enchanting voices, but sea monsters. In the sirens' episode, we could find *the natural position*, or the strength to cope with *the painful riddle of death* without consolatory answers but trying to confront truth just as Odysseus did.

The Greek hero becomes our travel partner when we decide, directly and naturally, to acknowledge uncertainty as well as paradox within our own life and also within our human condition, which determines us and is permanently present. Odysseus pleads with his men: "¡Please, untie me, untie me!." He was ready to confront in the most natural way *the painful riddle of death*. In the middle of that uncertainty and paradox, he returned to Ithaca.

Profound questions about the meaning of life live within all of us but they are questions that we could never answer beforehand. Odysseus found his answer as we are obliged to find our own. If answers were provided, uncertainty would be lost and we would be deceitfully connected with a kind of fullness ending in hollowness, emptiness and senselessness.

Here we would like to add another digression that can illustrate uncertainty and paradox. If we were to take certain punctuation marks, we would find the ones that corresponded to both. A colon (:), for example, opens its continuity to infinity and uncertainty; we could propose it as an example of the type of confrontation the maturescent individual is exposed to. In contrast, the ellipsis (...) only supposes continuity—known beforehand or inferred from what is being narrated—from this perspective, it could be considered as the antithesis of the colon. The former, on the other hand, suggests an abyss of meaning due to its unpredictability; this stance is the one proposed by maturescence when it invites subjectivity to the experience of uncertainty and paradox. Moreover, the colon leaves the road open for what exists beyond repetitive compulsion.

The tension between both components—paradox and uncertainty—can be found in the following paragraph, extracted from Freud's (August 13th, 1937) letter to Marie Bonaparte:

> The moment a man questions the meaning and value of life, he is sick, since objectively neither has any existence; by asking this question one is merely admitting to a store of unsatisfied libido to which something else must have happened, a kind of fermentation leading to sadness and depression.

Freud points out that at the same moment an individual questions the meaning of life he ends up losing it; in that instant, uncertainty and paradox disappear and defensive mechanisms are set in motion at the service of regression.

Continuing with this idea, the *meaning* of maturescence is something that makes evident the drive increase process that Freud posed. When this drive increase is set in motion, individuals experience the need to search for a meaning of what they are experiencing, as if they were trying to solve *the revolt against biology*. And this is the reason why the question about meaning of the (human) riddle of life and death is consciously raised during maturescence.

Psychic life is marvelous, psychic life is scarce; we suppose it only dwells in so called human beings. We must take care of and preserve psychic life but we will have a collective common future when we can understand where this psychic life comes from. This author's idea is that psychic life exists if we take nature into account and, as human beings, we cannot live as if we were not a part of nature. From this awareness, a different future for humanity is possible.

Uncertainty and clinical practice

How can we determine whether dealing with maturescence contributes to maturity (development and growth)? One could infer several indicators constituting the direct consequence of the (always relative) ways of dealing with the second moratorium (maturescence); one is central, the other four, subsidiary.

To integrate (acknowledge) uncertainty (*mors certa, hora incerta*) [certain death, uncertain time] implies working-through maturescence and is linked to the futility of existence (paradox) from a biological perspective and the transient nature of existence from a psychoanalytical perspective. This experience comes directly from the unconscious perception that the time remaining to live is intimately related to the second moratorium and its psychic effects.

Freud (1919h) connects uncertainty with the uncanny, which in full strength could lead to the extreme defenses that occur in maturescent crises because intolerance concerning uncertainty introduces the uncanny directly into psychic life, disrupting all psychic integration.

According to Freud:

> A particularly favourable condition for awakening uncanny feelings is created when there is intellectual uncertainty whether an object is alive or not, and when an inanimate object becomes too much like an animate one... We remember that in their early games children do not distinguish at all sharply between living and inanimate objects, and that they are especially fond of treating their dolls like live people.
>
> [p. 233]

The awareness of this tension between the animate and the inanimate, the unconscious omnipresence of childhood fantasies with respect to the secret life of objects, contributes to the experience of uncertainty.

In this regard, we would like to consider the work of the Russian philosopher Vladimir Yankélévitch (1903–1985) who maintains:

> If *mors certa, hora certa* is the formula of despair, *Mors certa, hora certa sed ignota* the formula of anguish and, conversely, *Mors incerta, hora incerta* the formula of chimerical hope, we should recognize in the dyssimetric formula *Mors certa, hora incerta* the emblem of a serious and militant will, as far removed from despair as chimeric hope.
>
> (1977) [p. 149]

It is very interesting to draw a parallel between what Yankélévitch points out and fundamental psychoanalytic meta-psychological tenets, since from a philosophical perspective it depicts some paths associated with the tension between certainty and uncertainty which this author has been referring to.

Yankélévitch suggests four paths resulting from the different combinations of both concepts. He therefore proposes four formulas: the formula of despair, the formula of anguish, the formula of chimeric hope and the formula of serious and militant will ... with life, equivalent to the natural position, as we have previously put forward. The reader will find a parallel with the equivalent paths proposed by Freud (1916a [1915]) in *On Transience*, where he identifies three possible dispositions that can arise in the face of the transitory (perishing), that is, in what is fated to disappear, as previously sustained in this chapter.

Clinical vignettes

The following vignettes evince the importance uncertainty has at the outset of maturescence as it unfolds. A successful professional aged 48, married and father of three children, comes to his therapy session terribly worried about "the country's situation," which he feels is becoming "hardly secure." Consequently, he has gradually shifted his assets out of the country so as to "ascertain his future" and that of his children. The interpretation that follows is an example of how one can integrate (acknowledge) uncertainty during maturescence's early days:

> I don't doubt that you can find a way to save your assets, but it seems to me that what you're telling me is deeper than that; perhaps a concern to find some place safe from the uncertainties of your adult life. Because when you talk about the "country's situation" you're actually talking about your situation as an adult, where you must handle an enormous amount of uncertainty every day. Likewise, you might also be alluding to the "situation in your analysis", where instead of offering you some consolation and tranquility, it makes you confront day in and day out a set of questions to formulate over and over again, questions that have no answer.

A 50-year-old actor, divorced and father of four children, has a tremendous "fear of flying". Furthermore, this fear is in direct conflict with his profession because it requires considerable air travel. He mentions the large amount of tranquilizers he takes when he travels. The session before a particular trip he arrives in an altered and anxious state. He begs his analyst to guarantee that the plane will not crash. The following is the interpretation the analyst offered to the patient from the vertex of his maturescence:

> I'm not going to tell you that you're overly scared because you yourself tell me this over and over again. But it seems to me that when you bring up your fear of flying, what you really want me to tell you is that you're

not going to die. And I cannot lie about that. Some day you're going to die, just like me and everybody else. I think that you ask for this in the same way one of your children might ask for reassurance concerning something he's afraid of. In your kids' case, they still need to believe that their father has the answers to all their problems and fears because they are still children. But you're a grown-up, I can't treat you like a child and lie to you saying the plane won't crash. In fact, sometimes planes do crash in mid-air. However, I think I can help you by not letting the "analytic airplane" crash. We can go on flying if you can acknowledge the natural uncertainty you inevitably must get used to because you are an adult.

It would seem that the reactions of these patients with respect to uncertainty are the clinical nucleus from which it is possible to work-through the onset of maturescence. These clinical vignettes imply, in the first case, a relative integration (acknowledgement) of uncertainty; and in the second case, given the obvious preoccupation with death, it is clear that such an integration has not occurred.

Clinical experience also indicates that, in many cases, whether the interpretation alludes to or not to the somatic source from which the demand of psychic work comes from is not essential, as the two clinical examples illustrate. Perhaps when it concerns the interpretation of dreams, as we will demonstrate in the chapter *The expression of maturescence in dreams*, the reference to a somatic source will become necessary. The interpretation from the paradox towards an experience of uncertainty implies a course from one's consciousness towards the unconscious; this necessarily includes a somatic source. We should note, therefore, that what does become essential for the psychoanalyst is to be well positioned, comprehending the somatic source from which the psychic work originates. Only then will he be able to find the opportunity and pertinence that will allow him to allude to the somatic.

Dealing with uncertainty

We should now consider what actually takes place in the analytic process because a psychoanalyst's own outlook concerning uncertainty is a key factor in order to accompany the patient in his strategy for dealing with uncertainty. These matters could be understood as *caesura* of uncertainty in maturescence. Bion suggests that *caesura* exists between patient and analyst and is pathognomonic of each analytic process. Through *caesura* (Bion, 1990) it is possible to invest or de-invest (often simultaneously) the uncertainty both patient and analyst are generating, so as to facilitate or inhibit the working-through process. At the same time, it would seem that *caesura* of uncertainty *is alive* and can permanently mutate its appearance and its trapping to the extent that patient and analyst confront uncertainty or retreat from it. As Kavka (2014) observes, we cannot treat the aging process but we can analyze aging individuals. In this respect, we would like to add that the analyst is also aging and is an active counterpart of the *caesura* during maturescence.

An analogue of maturescence can be also found in what Said (2006) has proposed concerning the *late style* in the literary or musical creation of many artists. Certain artists epitomize people who have managed to integrate (acknowledge) their experience of uncertainty in their creative productions. Their acknowledgement provides them with an opening that evinces an alternative personal commitment not controlled by the spirit of the time. It is an open question whether this *late style* is applicable to anybody's daily life rather than only to artists. This is a matter worth researching. At any rate, this proposal would seem to diverge from Jaques's conclusions in his classic study of the mid-life crisis, where he proposes that certain creative *styles* at that point in life depend on the Kleinian paranoid–schizoid position and on the depressive position. Clinical evidence seems to contradict Jaques's proposal, making it possible to find several different creative styles that are much closer to what Said describes.

On these grounds, we suggest that the integration (acknowledgement) of uncertainty and paradox are the clinical indicators par excellence of the working-through of the maturescent's drive increase. In this case, integration (acknowledgement) is in permanent tension with the implicit disintegration (rejection) associated with worries about death, provided that the individual is not threatened by a serious illness. In fact, someone who is afraid of getting old and of dying has stopped his development and growth. Once uncertainty and paradox have been integrated (acknowledged), people can concentrate on the experience of being alive. They can accept that growing old is part of nature even though it emerges as "the most touchy point in the narcissistic system" (Freud) (1914c) [p. 91].

While experiencing uncertainty and paradox, we can subsume an acknowledgement of our hatred and destructivity, directed at ourselves and at others, as inherent to human nature. Jaques (1965) was the first to identify that what he called the mid-life crisis also entails this recognition of hatred. It is a direct consequence of one's coping (relatively) with maturescence, which comes from the resurgence and re-working through of the Oedipal conflict. This acknowledgement also has a source in human nature's inherent affective ambivalence.

During maturescence, a change in the subjective perception of time can also take place, entailing a new and increased appreciation of the present. It simultaneously re-signifies the past and the future in their perpetual twofold conflict. This is an unfathomable experience subsumed in a circular and permanent process within the uncertainty of the present.

Another element deriving from experiencing uncertainty and paradox is related to a novel integration of the individual's life history. It allows the individual to resolve what Freud (1909c [1908]) called the family romance [p. 240] and his/her personal myth in a different fashion. In a similar way, Bollas

(1989) differentiates between fate and destiny, as was already mentioned in this chapter. He distinguishes their origins, purposes, and the transformation of fate into destiny, which could be considered intrinsic to maturescence. This is due to the compelling nature of phylogeny and extended biology that come into play during this moratorium.

As a consequence of integrating one's personal history in a different fashion, the next subsidiary element can be to anchor personal history in generational history, as Singman de Vogelfanger (2006) has proposed. This process would operate in two directions simultaneously. One vector points to the past, the other toward the future. The former entails a process that promotes a different acquisition of the familiar (generational) history. This perception is different from that of the generational conflict in all its variations. This generational transmission toward prior and subsequent generations is additional evidence that the maturescent moratorium is being managed.

These are the clinical pointers: one is central (uncertainty) the other four (acknowledgement of one's own hatred and destructivity, change of subjective perception of time, novel integration of the individual's life history, and anchor personal history in generational history), subsidiary. They contribute to the psychic working through (always relative) transformation that maturescence demands. The achievement of maturescence as development and growth leading to true maturity has a common denominator: the acknowledgement of and confrontation with uncertainty and paradox.

Chapter 3

The expression of maturescence in dreams

The working-through of maturescence can also be inferred through dreams; the latter offer the opportunity of detecting somatic processes that evince the magnitude of the psychic work generated by masculine and feminine climacterics—an unavoidable universal for all human beings. It is important to highlight an understanding of the somatic processes as related to biology and an understanding of bodily processes as related to psychology—the soma invested by drive activity.

An exegesis of the expression of maturescence present in dreams requires a definition of various vertexes:

a. The somatic source
b. The somatic nucleus
c. The *actual* factor

These three vertexes are essential for an interpretation of dreams that includes the working-through of maturescence as an additional level to the classic interpretation of wish fulfillment: the fulfillment of the unconscious wish of a never ending fertility.

The somatic source

As early as in *The Interpretation of Dreams* (1900a), Freud maintains that the internal (organic) corporal stimulus is one of the most important stimuli and as well as one of the most important sources of dreams:

> If it is established that the interior of the body when it is in a diseased state becomes a source of stimuli for dreams, and if we admit that during sleep the mind, being diverted from the external world, is able to pay more attention to the interior of the body, then it seems plausible to suppose that the internal organs do not need to be disabled before they can cause excitations to reach the sleeping mind—excitations which are somehow turned into dream-images. While we are awake we are aware of a diffuse general sensibility or coenaesthesia, but only as a vague quality

of our mood; to this feeling, according to medical opinion, all the organic systems contribute a share. At night, however, it would seem that this same feeling, grown into a powerful influence and acting through its various components, becomes the strongest and at the same time the commonest source for instigating dream-images.

[p. 35]

Here we find how the somatic source functions as one of the motors of dreams.

The somatic nucleus

Furthermore, the transcendence that Freud gives to the source of somatic stimuli can lead to the consideration of the dream's navel as the place (*topos*, in Greek; *locus*, in Latin) where the interface between the psychic and the somatic establishes a kind of frontier: that is the place where the regressive psychical processing which characterizes the work of dreams becomes truly rooted in the somatic. In the same book, Freud further sustains (1900a):

> There is often a passage in even the most thoroughly interpreted dream which has to be left obscure; this is because we become aware during the work of interpretation that at that point there is a tangle of dream-thoughts which cannot be unraveled and which moreover adds nothing to our knowledge of the content of the dream. This is the dream's navel, the spot where it reaches down into the unknown. The dream-thoughts to which we are led by interpretation cannot, from the nature of things, have any definite endings; they are bound to branch out in every direction into the intricate network of our world of thought. It is at some point where the meshwork is particularly close that the dream-wish grows up, like a mushroom out of its mycelium.

[p. 525]

The place where the unknown starts and from where the dream wish will emerge, then, is a space devoid of psychic representation, a fact which, precisely due to this lack, allows us to consider that the somatic root is always present in the formation of dreams. Perhaps for this reason, Freud also affirms:

> There is at least one spot in every dream at which it is unfathomable—a navel, as it were, that is its point of contact with the unknown.

[p. 111, f. 2]

This place of contact between sleep and the unknown functions also as its source. Moreover, if we can assume that it reaches down into the somatic, it would be imperative to consider the somatic processes as necessarily having their expression in sleep.

The *actual* factor

> Dreams admit of another and subtler interpretation, which in fact becomes unavoidable if we take a subsidiary detail into account. The two interpretations are not mutually contradictory, but both cover the same ground; they are a good instance of the fact that dreams, like all other psychopathological structures, regularly have more than one meaning.
>
> [p. 147]

With this assertion, Freud (1900a) opens a new dimension to this elaboration because it leads to the consideration of the actual question. All dreams have at least two levels of interpretation: the dream as a wish fulfillment—the traditional interpretation of dreams—and the dream as the expression of the *actual* situation, with all its implications—where the wish is also fulfilled, although in this case special emphasis is placed on the somatic factor.

These two levels of interpretation of the unconscious wish fulfillment in dreams distinguish the *body*—the soma invested with drive activity, the body of psychoanalysis—and the *soma*—the body of biology—where unconscious wish is also fulfilled although from a different level—as was mentioned at the beginning of this chapter. This last level is the one associated with the *actual*.

The problem generated by the translation of the concept of *actual* is worth considering. In English; *actual* is a more precise term, whereas in Spanish and other languages it becomes rather blurred. In the former, actual means real; in Spanish, however, it is less clear: (1) *present, at the same moment*; and (2) *that exists, happens or which is used at the time of speaking*.

Dreams, therefore, allow for an *actual* interpretation that can be a part of the interpretation of the wish fulfillment, although the interpretation can also be considered in two different levels: the interpretation at the level of wish and the interpretation at the actual level—both fulfill and point at the unconscious wish fulfillment.

Naturally when we consider the question of the *actual*, the Freudian concept that all psychoneurosis has a nucleus based on the actual neurosis resonates. Freud (1912f) affirms:

> My view is still what it was in the first instance, more than fifteen years ago: namely, that the ... "actual neurosis" provide the psychoneuroses with the necessary "somatic compliance" they provide the excitatory material, which is then psychically selected and given a "psychical coating," so that, speaking generally, the nucleus of the psychoneurotic symptom—the grain of sand in the centre of the pearl—is formed of a somatic sexual manifestation.
>
> [p. 248]

Freud (1905e [1901]) illustrates the Dora case with his famous metaphor:

In the lowest stratum we must assume the presence of a real and organic-ally determined irritation ... which acted like the grain of sand around which an oyster forms its pearl.

[p. 83]

From this perspective, it is possible to discover, as an integral part of the dream manifestation, the existence of a grain of sand that metaphorizes the somatic source present in all dreams.

Summary of the three vertexes

In summary, we can refer to a source, a nucleus and a factor in order to com-prehend the somatic processes activated during climacterics in men and women:

1. A *somatic source* exists for the genesis of dreams.
2. A *somatic nucleus* exists which could represent an equivalent of the navel of dreams—a *place* where representations merge with the somatic.
3. An *actual factor* exists which is necessary for the formation of dreams—equivalent to the *actual* factor (*real*, different from psychic, in this case) present in all neuroses.

These three factors allow us to infer—in conjunction with the work of inter-pretation of dreams during a psychoanalytic session—that the somatic phenom-ena present in the peri-climacteric processes in men and women have their expression in dream formation and are liable to interpretation.

The *pretty butcher's wife's* dream (also known as the smoked *salmon*'s dream)

Freud (1900a) quotes *the pretty butcher's wife's dream* (*smoked salmon*) in *The Interpretation of Dreams* [pp. 146–150], holding that the patient made refer-ence to it in an attempt to contradict the theory that dreams always imply a wish fulfillment:

> You're always saying to me ... that a dream is a fulfilled wish. Well, I'll tell you a dream whose subject was the exact opposite—a dream in which one of my wishes was *not* fulfilled. How do you fit that in with your theory?
>
> [p. 146]

She would seem more like someone who asked a question rather than a patient in an analysis session. For this reason, we will refer to her as the *dreamer* rather than a *patient*, in spite of Freud's assertion of her as his patient. And she described the following dream:

I wanted to give a supper-party, but I had nothing in the house but a little smoked salmon. I thought I would go out and buy something, but remembered then that it was Sunday afternoon and all the shops would be shut. Next I tried to ring up some caterers, but the telephone was out of order. So I had to abandon my wish to give a supper-party.

[p. 147]

As usual—as the first step towards the interpretation of dreams and before any associations—Freud asked her what she had done the day before:

As you know, the instigation to a dream is always to be found in the events of the previous day.

[p. 147]

The dreamer then related that her husband, "an honest and capable wholesale butcher" [p. 147], had mentioned to her that since he was getting fat, he wanted to start a diet in order to lose weight. He told her that he would get up early, do exercise, diet, and especially, that he would not accept dinner invitations. He also told her, laughing, that the day before he had met an artist who wanted "to paint his portrait as he had never seen such expressive features" [p. 147]. The husband, however had refused the offer because "... he was sure the painter would prefer a piece of a pretty young girl's behind to the whole of his face" [p. 147]. Furthermore, the patient affirms she is in love with her husband and that she likes to joke with him:

She had begged him, too, not to give her any caviar.

[p. 147]

Freud interrupts her to ask her what she had meant with respect to the caviar. The patient answers that for a long time she had wanted to have some caviar before lunch "but had grudged the expense." [p. 147]. She knows that if she asked her husband, he would immediately obtain it for her but she begged him not to give her any so that she could continue to tease him about it.

After a pause, Freud states that the patient comments that on the previous day she had gone to visit a friend:

The day before she had visited a woman friend of whom she confessed she felt jealous because her (my patient's) husband was constantly singing her praises.

[p. 148]

She is not worried, however because "fortunately this friend of hers is very skinny and thin and her husband admires a plumper figure" [p. 148]. They had both chatted about the friend's wish to "to grow a little stouter" [p. 148] and her hope that she would be invited once again to supper:

You always feed one so well.

[p. 148]

Freud then interprets that the wish that she fulfills with her dream is not inviting her friend to supper so that the latter will not be able to obtain a plumper figure, and therefore become more attractive to her husband. In that case, the patient replies:

I'd rather never give another supper-party.

[p. 148]

But Freud realizes that something else is needed that will confirm his interpretation. He therefore asks her about the smoked salmon. The patient replies:

Smoked salmon is my friend's favourite dish.

[p. 148]

Freud then adds that the dreamer's wish acquires a second meaning, if regarded as the patient's wish that her friend will not achieve her wish-fulfillment of gaining some weight. Consequently, instead of dreaming that her friend will not achieve her wish-fulfillment, she dreams that she herself does not fulfill her own wish:

But instead of this she dreamt that one of her *own* wishes was not fulfilled.

[p. 148]

Finally, Freud asserts that the dream allows for an understanding of the processes of hysterical identification:

My patient put herself in her friend's place in the dream because her friend was taking my patient's place with her husband and because she (my patient) wanted to take her friend's place in her husband's high opinion.

[p. 150]

Interpretation of the pretty butcher's wife's dream from the perspective of maturescence

As anticipated, the dream is a psychic process that allows an interpretation which will integrate the somatic processes, since these can be considered a level of expression present in all dreams and their interpretation. This level does not invalidate other levels of interpretation, particularly the one that has to do with the conception of dreams as a traditional wish fulfillment but, rather, it integrates them.

If we consider that the specific processes of maturescence also take place in dreams, this level of interpretation can be centered in the dream work that accounts for that which is expressed as a result of and during maturescence, transforming itself in an exclusive psychic phenomenon where both perspectives are simultaneously present.

It has already been established that the soma is an *actual* factor, present in all dreams. For this reason, the *place* where dreams take place makes a precise reference to the dreamer's own soma—not only to the body. The actual somatic state appears represented in the dream scenario, providing indications of its functioning and eventual alterations. Somehow or other, the dream implies both a continent and a somatic content which demands an interpretation that accompanies and deepens the classic interpretation of wish fulfillment.

In the interpretation of the pretty butcher's wife's dream, which will be presented from this perspective, it is necessary to highlight the quality of applied psychoanalysis it contains—the attempt could be taken as an example of wild analysis *per via de porre*—since none of the conditions that make an interpretation reliable exist: the physical presence of the patient in the session, the transferential situation and the contra-transferential register, the spontaneity of the associations, the moment during the session chosen for the description of the dream, previous associations of the dream and so many other factors which are essential for the interpretation of a dream in all psychoanalytic treatments. It is only a clinical exercise, to which an example of an ongoing treatment will be subsequently added where the same type of interpretation will be detailed.

It is also important to point out that it was impossible to find references of the real butcher's wife, despite efforts from scholars dedicated to identifying Freud's patients; no one had any information regarding this patient. The lack of any records of the patient's identity seemed indeed very odd, considering the quantity of patients treated by Freud whose identities were finally revealed. The ambition of the search, therefore, was to find some reference related to age or health of the patient in order to have an added element to the interpretation provided below.

This author also wants to point out that Freud (1900a) is also interested in the representation of age in dreams. He mentions the subject many times [p. 409] [p. 416] [p. 437] [p. 512]. The reader can find several of these assumptions and comments in Chapter 7.

But at this stage it is important to quote the dream as it appears in Freud's text:

> I wanted to give a supper-party, *but* I had nothing in the house but a little smoked salmon. I thought I would go out and buy something, *but* remembered then that it was Sunday afternoon and all the shops would be shut.

Next I tried to ring up some caterers, *but* the telephone was out of order. So I had to abandon my wish to give a supper-party.

(Freud, 1900a) [p. 147]

It is surprising that Freud apparently did not consider the patient's insistence on the word *but*—there's no mention to it in the Freudian text—repeated three times during the brief account of her dream. This first level of analysis—which could be termed structural—provides us with some elements related to the dynamics of the psyche.

Grammatically, *but* is a coordinating conjunction whose function is to connect words, phrases or independent clauses. The conjunction *but*, however is always binary and is used to indicate contrast. It establishes a tension indicating a type of psychic functioning from which an interdiction of desire could be deduced. So far, this would be consistent with the dreamer's idea:

You're always saying to me ... that a dream is a fulfilled wish. Well, I'll tell you a dream whose subject was the exact opposite—a dream in which one of my wishes was *not* fulfilled. How do you fit that in with your theory?

[p. 146]

It is as if the dreamer were expressing her wish in several attempts and the same wish found itself restrained by a contrary motion—from the dreamer's perspective, she is authentically expressing what she feels.

Somehow, the frequent use of *but* while narrating her dream would express the reality of a wish that presses with force, since it barges in three times in one formulation despite her permanent rejection. What is that wish?

Note that the three beginning sentences: "give a supper-party," "go out and buy something," "ring up some caterers" make the wish evident; whereas the closing ones: "I had nothing in the house but a little smoked salmon," "[I] remembered then that it was Sunday afternoon and all the shops would be shut," and "the telephone was out of order" make evident the contrary motion to the desire referred to earlier.

What might one think if the dream was considered from the perspective of somatic processes? What would be the *but* expressed by the dreamer's soma?

In this context, the answer alludes to a simple hypothesis, raising this, of course, as an exercise of applied psychoanalysis. The dreamer is worried because she is commencing a menopausal process—in this case, it is immaterial for the unconscious whether the person has had children or not. Since it was not possible to obtain information about the real patient, as was previously mentioned, the analysis of the dream would lead to the presumption that it refers to a middle aged woman, a fact which is evident in the three starting sentences of interdiction of the wish:

1. "I had nothing in the house but a little smoked salmon"
2. "[I] remembered then that it was Sunday afternoon and all the shops would be shut"
3. "the telephone was out of order"

These three factors would force her to "abandon my wish to give a supper-party." That is to say: of having a child or knowing that she is still fertile?

As previously mentioned, the somatic *place* where the dreams take place allows us to comprehend that *the house, the shops* and *the telephone out of order* alluded to by the dreamer could indicate an *actual* representation of the soma; the uterus in this case, presumably incapable of continuing to house ova (uterus as house?)

Please note the starting sentences:

1. "give a supper-party"
2. "go out and buy something"
3. "ring up some caterers"

These three elements can serve as representation of the wish: becoming pregnant, if considered at the *somatic* level (but being desired as a woman at the *bodily* level). This can refer to a frequent fact activated during menopause: the difficulty of giving up the reproductive function, a natural and unavoidable occurrence of maturescence, let's say: the wish of a never ending fertility.

When the dreamer affirms: "I had to abandon my wish to give a supper-party," we can infer from the statement of obligation "had to" that something occurs against her wish; an induced situation, such as the menopausal mandate, imposes a law that cannot be modified.

It is difficult to establish the connotations of giving a supper-party. However, "ring up some caterers" could indicate not only the wish to be sexually invested by her husband but also being fertilized. A caterer is someone who provides that which we do not have; in this case, the spermatozoa that could fertilize her, thus attempting to nullify the anguish characteristic of menopause at the maturescent stage of life.

Likewise, "give a supper-party" could be recognized as the process of pregnancy and childbirth. But the dreamer states: "So I had to abandon my wish to give a supper-party," which would prompt the question: Isn't it possible to think that the desire which had to be relinquished is precisely the desire to become pregnant?

Something equivalent could be maintained with regard to gaining weight, if considered in the local slang that "having a bun in the oven" is used as an understatement for *pregnancy*. In fact, we could consider that the dreamer would have liked to become pregnant, although she knows she can't; her friend, on the other hand, could probably do so. Moreover, things could, in fact, be worse. The friend could become pregnant with the dreamer's husband, who seems to be physically capable of doing so, being "an honest and capable wholesale butcher" with such "such expressive features."

We could also consider this transferentially: when the dreamer challenges Freud with a dream that would contradict his theory of wish fulfillment, she would be asking him to make her pregnant, confirming her wish of being fertile by means of an interpretative and assisted fertilization that would contradict what she fears.

The theme of the salmon and the caviar also offers resonances linked to this subject. Salmon is a species of fish that at breeding time leaves open waters and migrates up river against the current. Many die in this process and those which do not, often cannot return. Could it be possible that in the dreamer's case, she wishes to deny the infertility mandate characteristic of menopause? Caviar, on the other hand, is the ova of the sturgeon fish. Both elements, salmon and caviar, therefore, allude to reproduction, with the nuance that caviar can also refer to the female ovaries; and we know that when the latter cease to function, menopause commences.

The dream of a patient in analysis

In the same way that we anticipated the quality of applied psychoanalysis to the pretty butcher's wife's dream, the dream described below, in contrast, meets all the formal requirements of an authentic dream because it was dreamt by an analytic patient in a transferential situation and was told during therapy. Then, the patient also was able to comment on the day's residues and the associations that arose at the time of narration. These facts and many other characteristics make this dream especially appropriate for the consideration of maturescence.

The case involves a patient who at the time of the dream was fifty-one years old and had previously attended therapy with this author during five years. Suddenly, she began to acknowledge a feeling of irritation, depression and discomfort, not knowing how to continue with her life. These feelings had been the same ones which had taken hold of her subjectivity when she was forty-six years old and had consulted for psychotherapy for the first time.

With two weekly sessions of psychoanalysis from the very beginning of psychotherapy, she had managed to stabilize her emotional state, sufficiently to partly resolve the mourning caused by her recent separation with her husband. The latter had suddenly left her for a younger woman, a fact which had consciously motivated her to look for psychotherapy. Moreover, the patient had had a son with her ex-husband, at the moment a young pre-adolescent. Since her separation, she had not fallen in love again and had only maintained casual relationships.

The patient's state of mind began to change as the psychoanalytic working-through progressed. This occurred in a satisfactory manner both for the patient and the analyst, with sessions that took place in relative calm and commitment despite the fact that in the weeks previous to the dream that will be related below, the patient felt once again the anguished emotional state that had led her to seek the assistance of a therapist.

In a session previous to the annual holidays of her sessions, she related the following dream:

> I saw myself at my ex-husband's wedding. He was with his wife and I was taking photographs of them. At one stage, I realized that I had run out of film. Nevertheless, I continued to take photos, even though I knew I had no more film left. I kept on trying despite feeling odd and obsessed with wanting to take more and more photos; this worried me, leaving me with a sense of not understanding what was happening to me.

The analyst found it significant that the patient mentioned feeling irritated and depressed when she narrated her dream. These emotional states were the same which she had grappled with during the weeks previous to the dream, although now they seemed their natural result. She was vexed because she felt like someone with only one thought in her mind, which she had to permanently wrestle with: the coming wedding of her ex-husband with a much younger woman, someone who had caused her separation—in her sayings. The sessions had already helped the patient discover that more than the age difference between her ex-husband and his new girlfriend, what really worried her was the actual difference between herself and the ex-husband's girlfriend, something qualitatively different for her subjectivity. However, even though this was something she was already aware of and thought she had overcome, that situation seemed to recur, in this case through the dream.

The emotional state occasioned by the oncoming wedding had been exhaustively dealt with during previous psychoanalytic sessions, reason why the factual circumstance that the wedding was soon to take place only added an *actual* nuance to a situation that seemed internally solved. It did not escape the psychoanalyst's attention, of course, that the manifested description of the dream was only that: an indicator that could lead to authentic dream thoughts. For this reason, the analyst knew that the associations would probably lead the interpretation to a different destiny, divergent from the wedding itself.

Regarding the day's residues, she commented that in previous days, while she waited for public transport to return home from work, she had seen a photography shop. She thought that it would be interesting if her only male son would become a photographer when he grew up. She believed it was an ageless profession because with it one did not become old and it was possible to maintain it for the rest of one's life. It is worth noting that the day's residues in this case also functioned as an association of the dream. As an added value, photography was related to art, one of her main interests.

After questioning the patient regarding the day's residues and asking her for associations, she maintained that her ex-husband's wedding really worried her because it was about to take place during the following weeks; this somehow contradicted everything that had been elaborated during the previous months. Furthermore, she stated that she had her eye on the wedding, wondering how it would all turn out. She also imagined that her son was not telling her all he knew about his father's wedding and his current situation, although she understood his silence and discretion. Furthermore, she attributed her wish to take photographs as a way of spying on her ex-husband in his new condition, since she thought she could not forgive the treason and abandonment, even though the psychoanalytic sessions had made her feel the opposite.

In addition, she related the effort she had made in the dream to take the photos and the anguish she felt when she realized they did not come out. By means of associations made by the patient, the analysis of the dream revealed that the camera left with no film were her ovaries without eggs. No matter how she tried, the fact remained that she was being left without eggs (film negatives) to take; they did not come out.

The emphasis on the verb take in the dream's narrative was also paradigmatic. The situation was different for her ex-husband, in the subjectivity of the patient. He could marry a younger woman, who still had film (eggs) to take photographs (was fertile), and together they could still have children, something off-limits for the patient. This was not due to the fact that she was no longer married to him but because nature had begun to make it difficult, thus initiating a period in her life which lacked previous representations (photographs). In this case, the photos were interpreted as attempts of representation of peri-menopausal reality, to which the patient was adapting.

A work of dream interpretation by levels can consider and include the experience of abandonment that the patient felt she was exposed to, the pain for what she had lost because of the separation, an interpretation of the primal scene, etc. However, from the perspective of the maturescent processes, the interpretation of the dream could consider that the wish she fulfilled with the dream was to remain fertile, whatever the cost, even though she also expressed the pain of knowing that she was being left without eggs (film); something that could also be understood from the fantasy of photography as an ageless profession because it did not age with her, among other various indicators of the wish for an everlasting fertility.

Transferentially, the patient would be asking her psychoanalyst for a representation of that which she cannot have because it can represent at the bodily level what happens with her peri-menopause—also understood as the concern for the lack of sexual desire: the fear to stop desiring and being desired: aphanisis as the underlying hidden side of drive increase—but it can hardly represent that which is linked at the somatic level—the wish of being always fertile—which explains the uncertainty of her emotional states as reflected in her worries and confusion.

Chapter 4

Nymphomaniac despair

Lolita (1955), the novel by Vladimir Nabokov (1899–1977), is the frequent arche-type of the love, passion and despair of the maturescent male for pubescent females. We consider it therefore appropriate for a psychoanalytic research on maturescence: what can lead an adult to fall hopelessly in love with a young adolescent? This inter-pretation hopes to find the causes that insist on desiring a relationship of this kind—quite a frequent phenomenon—and which can be considered related to the experi-ences characteristic of a certain type of maturescent course.

The novel was seriously distorted by its content, since it is usually associated with a genre that could be termed erotic/pseudo-pornographic, when, in fact, it portrays a profoundly existential and human drama. In part, this popular misrepre-sentation could be attributed to two movies which, somehow or other, modified the original theme, giving it an additional fame in extra-literary circles. Neverthe-less, the enormous impact caused by the publication of the novel cannot be under-estimated. Be that as it may, an insightful reader will undoubtedly rescue the true content of the work if it is approached without prejudice.

Nabokov was born in Saint Petersburg, into a wealthy Russian family. He had a privileged childhood that allowed him to learn Russian, English and French. His problems arose when he was eighteen years old, with the outbreak of the Bol-shevik Revolution in 1917, when the family had to abandon their home. Believing that they could remain in hiding for a brief time, they resorted to friends in Crimea, but two years later they fled to Europe. Vladimir studied languages in London and later established himself in Berlin in 1923 where, a year before, his father had been assassinated by mistake when he tried to protect a leader of the opposition. Two years later, he married Vera, his lifelong wife, with whom he had a son in 1934. He remained in Germany until 1937, when he moved to Paris. But in 1940 he decided to migrate to the United States due to the advance of German troops during the Second World War.

From his Berlin years, Nabokov distinguished himself as a novelist and poet and, once in America, he began to publish his works in English, earning his livelihood by teaching comparative literature, Russian and Russian literature courses at universities. In 1945, he obtained American citizenship.

Nabokov had three remarkable interests, which he enjoyed in his free time. Together with Vera, they had the amazing ability of synesthesia, attributing a color to each letter of the alphabet. The writer transferred this perceptual phenomenon to some of his characters. In addition, he was an expert entomologist, particularly of Lepidoptera, writing scientific papers on butterflies. He also conveyed this interest to some of his characters. Finally, he enjoyed composing chess problems, spending considerable time to make these problems more subtle and complex.

In 1953, Nabokov and his family travelled to Oregon, where he finished *Lolita*. The novel's enormous success, took him back to Europe in 1960, where he dedicated himself entirely to literature. He lived in Switzerland, in a hotel in Montreux until his death in 1977.

The novel commences with a prologue which explains that the author has died in prison, a few days before his trial for murder will begin. He has left a complete confession of his crime to the members of the jury. To gain credibility, the prologue maintains that the lawyer for the defendant has decided to deliver the document wherein the assassin narrates the story of his life, providing details of what led him to commit the crime. He also stresses that he has chosen to maintain the culprit's privacy, providing a pseudonym so as not to damage the reputation of those he has alluded to, in case the latter could be identified by eventual readers. His name will therefore be Humbert Humbert, or simply HH, throughout the text. From the beginning, therefore, the reader is uncertain as to who has been murdered by HH, a fact which will be revealed towards the end of the novel and which Nabokov handles with masterful skill.

The narration itself begins with a deep and open praise for his Lolita. Then, HH provides details of his childhood and narrates how his mother died by a lightning strike when he was three years old, although he hardly remembers her. His father, in turn, spoiled him a great deal, spending a lot of time with him. HH was proud of his father when he used to hear comments by the servants regarding his father's sentimental relationships. Furthermore at the beginning of the novel, HH confesses that Lolita had a precursor in his own childhood. Indeed, according to HH, Lolita might have never existed if it had not been for an early love. Annabel Leigh, the child referred to, was a few months older than HH and they both fell shamelessly in love.

HH describes in detail the ups and downs of his intense desire for Annabel, the ploys used to meet her in order to share brief physical encounters and her tragic death caused by typhus four months after he had met her. HH believes that Annabel's death left two important marks in his life. The first one, that Annabel was a true precursor of Lolita; and the second, that Annabel's unexpected death could have been the cause of his difficulty to fall in love, which he experienced throughout his youth, lamenting that Lolita had never loved him as his childhood sweetheart had.

Scholars of Nabokov's novel maintain that Annabel Leigh's name is an intertextual reference to Edgar Allan Poe's famous poem Annabel Lee. This is quite possible, since other references to the poem can be found throughout the work.

Nabokov, in fact, draws other similarities between HH's love for Lolita and other famous literary love relationships, including examples of courtly love. For example, the love of Dante Alighieri (1265–1321) for Beatrice Portinari, whom he had met when he was nine years old. Apparently, other than casual greetings on the street, the Italian poet never had a personal conversation with Beatrice or anything close to a true relationship. When she died, Dante took her as his model of beauty and supreme wisdom and she became a character of his *Divine Comedy* and *Vita Nuova*. These works reflect something enduring, equivalent, according to the author of *Lolita*, to HH's feelings for Annabel, although in Dante's case there was no such age difference.

Nabokov also mentions that Petrarch (1304–1374) experienced a similar infatuation for his Laura. Even though the Renaissance poet was about twenty years old when he met Laura, he did not have personal contact with her. Apparently, she was married and could therefore not accept him. Possibly due to her elusiveness, his love for her is an expression of immense joy and lasting desire. Neither was there an age difference in this case, so notable in the case of HH and Lolita. Would this be another ploy by the author to mislead the reader?

Finally, Nabokov makes reference to Poe's great love for Virginia Clemm, his first cousin. The latter was fourteen years old when she married the writer, who was then twenty-seven. A few years after their marriage, Virginia had the first symptoms of tuberculosis and died five years later. Poe was deeply affected by his wife's death, which led him to excessive drinking that eventually made him emotionally unstable. He died only two years after Virginia passed away.

By way of digression, this author would also like to add a famous criminal case that took place in 1948 in the United States involving the abduction of the eleven-year-old girl, Florence Horner. Her fifty-year-old kidnapper, Frank La Salle, discovered her stealing an item of small value but used this as a pretext to kidnap the child, taking her on a twenty-month trip around several states, with the permanent threat of revealing her misdemeanor. This famous case, which shocked public opinion, could have served Nabokov as a basis for *Lolita*'s main plot.

Further research on the novel has also suggested that the writer could have suffered from cryptomnesia, when a forgotten memory returns without it being recognized as such, thus using a plot similar to what had been previously written. In fact, Heinz von Lichberg had written his novel *Lolita* in 1916. The plot deals with an older man who becomes obsessed with a pre-adolescent also called Lolita that results in a long and never-ending trip. The book was published before Nabokov lived in Germany and had great success. All the same, the "factual" version and the "cryptomnesic" version in no way tarnish the merit of Nabokov's novel.

The examples of Annabel in the novel we are discussing and those of Poe, Dante and Petrarch evince intense loves—prohibited or incestuous—that function as initiatory relationships, often culminating in the death of the woman concerned. In many of these cases, as it occurs with HH in *Lolita*, this is manifested as an irrepressible and painful desire, made evident with great clarity and narrated in a powerful emotional tone. These situations, however, always remain frozen in time, highlighting the difficulty of psychic elaboration and allowing the reader to perceive how the main character tries to avoid a collapse within himself.

This collapse would allude to a certain experience of death—drive increase confronted with the background of the underlying aphanisis. This *death* could be understood as representing certain ends related to the passage of time and the different vicissitudes experienced at the conscious psychic level, together with the need of working-through maturescent drive increase and the profound void caused by aphanisis, both starting with maturescence as the forthcoming stage of life.

This despair—the effort to represent, or the discharge towards action, when representation is no longer possible—can be interpreted as an attempt to hang onto life. Moreover, this terror of collapse has to do with the perception and the difficulty to acknowledge individual's own aging, something consciously perceived by many people as an anticipation of death.

HH describes his passion for pubescent girls, particularly between the age of nine and fourteen, describing them as inhuman or demoniacal and referring to them as *nymphets*. *Nymphomaniacs*, therefore, would be men desperate to find girls who possessed this bewitching effect, in order to live a private passion with them; in this case, a subjective, unknown, passion for a nymphet as well as an objective, shared passion.

The characteristic of *nymphets* is that they can suddenly awaken the erotic desire of a man in an unrenounceable manner, since girls who possess this special charm makes them completely desirable. HH considers himself an expert in their detection. The relationship between a *nymphet* and a male adult is inversely proportional to the irruption of adolescent sexuality (drive increase and first moratorium) and the commencement of the maturescent somatic collapse (drive increase and second moratorium), both stemming from the same somatic source although with contrary valencies, as was mentioned in Chapter 2.

What takes place is an activation of the tension between maturescent drive increase and the fear of loss of individual's own erogeneity and eroticism—manifested as the subjective perception, recognized or not, of individual's own aging. In some people, this fear is *softened* by the reaffirmation provided by the presence of someone who is beginning to live this same erogeneity and eroticism drive increased but feared to be lost through aphanisis, thus establishing an *equilibrium*, although inversely proportional, as it was already mentioned. The formula implies that the more HH fears losing this kind of vitality, the more he needs to balance it with these *nymphomanic* presences.

We should consider that what apparently excites a *nymphomaniac* male is the incipient eroticism of the pubescent girl—something which could be considered as an unconscious perception of infertility (soma) and the uprising and collapse of desires (body). For this reason, it is not surprising that the condition for detecting the state of a *nymphet* is only privy to really older men, as Nabokov describes it. Faced with the subjective awareness of their own aging—or denying it through the veils of drive increase—certain maturescent men would need the reassurance implied in knowing that they can rely on the young body of a *nymphet*. Thus, they remain under the illusion that they are not losing the eroticism and potency they wish to retain, perhaps as an expression of an also illusory search for a certain kind of *immortality*.

HH describes how he has lived a dissociated adult life: a public life, where he has always tried to keep up appearances of normality, and a private one in which he desperately attempted to associate himself with different *nymphets* in order to keep his secret passion for each of them alive. He also affirms that he could provide a long list of some *unilateral* romances to demonstrate the intensity of his desire and the despair implied in such a quest.

This symptom implies the need to maintain a form of eroticism alive, raising once again the problem of its possible disappearance. It would seem that HH is afraid to lose something of himself if he does not re-encounter the passion that *nymphets* awaken in him. What could he be afraid of losing? Once again, aphanisis provides the answer. In addition, HH seems to confront an internal and intense vacuum and the close presence of a *nymphet* serves to counter that feeling of emptiness. What HH considers eroticism could be translated with the word *life*. In this respect, he would be fearing the loss of his own personal integration, his experience of being himself, every time he does not have a *nymphet* close by, especially someone like Lolita, as his guarantee of *immortality*.

Of course, this symptomatology occurs to people who are predisposed to maintain such a course due to specific historical and personal circumstances. Nymphomania is usually perceived as a fantasy, although *extreme cases* like the ones expressed by HH usually help to understand in depth the *common cases*, where everything takes place within the limits of fantasy. Neither do we forget that HH's *clinical case* is a literary work that serves as a basis to analyze one type, among many others, of the maturescent process.

HH was married for a few years. His marriage, however, was a wretched one because he had not searched for a loving wife. Neither had he married her for her beauty but rather for a companion that could help him to control his desires, or at least to calm them down. Soon after the wedding, he felt that his wife was turning into a despicable person, just like his mother, and he decided to separate. Another factor which led to the separation was the news that his American uncle had made him his heir, with the condition that he should settle in the United States. He therefore suggests to his wife the need to emigrate, hoping that she will refuse. His spouse confesses that she has been involved with someone else for some time and prefers to remain, thus encouraging the separation.

Soon after his arrival to the United States, HH has to be repeatedly confined to psychiatric institutions due to nervous exhaustion, melancholic crises and violent outbursts of anxiety. In between, he visits Arctic Canada, trying to find tranquility among the Eskimos. However, this proves to be a fiasco, since he is unable to find a *nymphet* among the Eskimo women.

At this juncture, an employee of his late uncle suggests to him a trip to the countryside, since he has some friends who could provide him with lodgings. They have two children: a baby and a twelve-year-old daughter. HH is immediately attracted to the idea of finding a *nymphet* in this child and recuperates his enthusiasm and lost hope. However, on the day that he was to arrive at the town hotel in order to resume his journey the next morning, his uncle's ex-employee informs him that the cottage where he was to be lodged has burnt down. Nevertheless, he offers him alternative accommodation at the house of a widow, Clara Haze, who also has a twelve-year-old daughter as well as a room to let. Upon arrival to his new lodgings, HH feels he has had a revelation: When he sees the girl, he experiences a flashback of his childhood sweetheart: the same fragility, chestnut hair and supple skin, the juvenile breasts he had fondled as a young boy but now contemplated with his aging eyes, as if the twenty-five years that had elapsed had vanished in one instant.

Thus he discovers Lolita, who now represents his lost Annabel. From now on, HH will remain completely infatuated. Lolita finds a reinforcement in the previous affective history of the protagonist; she is herself, but recharged with the force Annabel had. HH's difficulty for separations and mourning processes is notorious, as if he had never been able to solve what had been left pending with Annabel. And we therefore ask: what would have been HH's life course if Annabel had not died? In any event, Annabel brings to the forefront what HH has experienced traumatically. This unresolved issue remains adhered to the person of Lolita.

In this way the theme of maturescence reappears. HH has searched all his life for someone who could substitute Annabel but only *finds* it in his maturescence. In this case, it could be considered that the typical drive increase is what leads him to the object, establishing the relationship. He then commences to describe the ploys he makes up to produce *casual* encounters with Lolita that can lead to physical contact: placing his hand on her lap, sitting her on his knees, masturbating against her body, each day with more desperation, greater intimacy, each instant with a renewed need. At the same time, being a man with literary interests, he writes about his emotional experiences in a secret diary where he records his feelings and his disinterest for Clara, her mother.

Clara, on the other hand, seeks his aid in rearing Lolita, expressing her concern that her daughter might take the wrong path in life. For this reason, she has taken the decision to send her to a summer camp for several weeks, a situation that depresses him deeply. Soon afterwards, she gives him a letter confessing her love for him and asking him to marry her. In case of refusal, he must leave immediately. She also expresses her wish that he will become a father to her daughter. This makes HH very happy, since once in this position, he can be in daily reach of Lolita's caresses. He then speculates on the series of opportunities that would arise with his *daughter*. He daydreams of administering a sleeping pill to his new wife in order to caress Lolita all night with impunity. He also imagines Clara pregnant because a Cesarean delivery would allow him to be alone with Lolita for several days, and even considers administering Lolita herself with a sleeping pill, obviously with sexual intentions.

At this point the reader can consider two fundamental interests expressed by HH. On the one hand, the fulfillment of his sexual desire for Lolita and, on the other, the expression of a series of fantasies regarding what it means to have a child. But the intensity is provided by the despair he feels to sexually possess Lolita; the desire that hides his need of Lolita as something that connects him with life. And here the word *need* appears: HH "needs" Lolita. Due to this need, we can regard Lolita's presence as something that would function as a non-pharmacological *antidepressant*. Since HH needs Lolita, he imagines extreme *solutions*: bringing about Clara's death in order to remain Lolita's *guardian*.

Since Clara is truly worried about her daughter and is, at the same time, profoundly jealous of the growing reciprocity between her daughter and HH, she decides to send her to a boarding school for young girls. As a result, HH feels that the only possible solution is to kill Clara. He begins to imagine a way of doing so without raising suspicion, although he is concerned about the sense of guilt he would harbor for the rest of his life.

Chronic jealousy makes Clara inquisitive regarding HH's past until she finally discovers his diary. Desperate and disappointed, she confronts HH, who tries to defend himself by explaining that the diary is only the draft of a future novel and the names only coincidences. He tries to calm her and fetches two whisky glasses but, while he does so, a neighbor telephones him to say that Clara has just been run over by a car. Initially, HH cannot believe it, insisting that it cannot be true, since his wife had been with him only a moment ago. However, he immediately confirms that Clara has left and is, in fact, the person who has just died.

That night HH gets drunk in order to sleep soundly—satisfied—and the next day he feels ready to enjoy the social permission everyone has granted him to take care of the orphan Lolita. He imagines her crying on his shoulder and pressing herself against him, in search of that yearned pleasure that her contact will give him. He would be an exemplary father and would rescue Lolita from her grief. From then onwards, he considers he has arrived at a climax; he would possess *his* Lolita forever, almost as if he had been able to detain time.

However, after Clara's burial, HH changes plans. He figures that it would be better to take Lolita away from the boarding school, with the excuse that his mother was about to undergo an important operation. He would begin to travel with Lolita, moving from one hotel to another until he would finally let her know of her mother's death. When he goes to fetch her and tells her that he has missed her, Lolita answers that she had not; what is more, she has been shamelessly disloyal. She then proceeds to throw herself into his arms and, despite his initial coyness, she presses her lips against his, making him feel her front teeth and taste her mint-flavored saliva.

At the first hotel they arrive at, HH requests a room with an extra bed for his twelve-year-old daughter, who is very tired. Once in the room, HH tells her that he will sleep in the extra bed but immediately the conversation reaches its climax. HH tells her that, in her mother's absence, he is responsible for her and they must get used to sharing this kind of intimacy. Lolita, on the other hand, tells him that what they were about to experience had only one name: incest.

Even though he had previously decided to give her a sleeping pill so that she would not realize his intentions, fifteen minutes later they had their first sexual encounter. Moreover, HH is surprised by the fact that it was Lolita who seduced him, rather than the other way around, thus fulfilling a lifelong dream.

Instead of satisfying him, this first sexual encounter disturbs HH to the point where he feels it has surpassed its mark, turning into a nightmare, awakening instead an insatiable desire for Lolita, now a *miserable nymphet*.

What disturbs him even more is that Lolita displays an autonomy and liberty he had not previously noticed. Once again the theme of aging appears. Lolita acts like a woman profoundly interested in the pleasures of the body, acknowledging the difference obtained in each one. She also surprises him by confessing that she is not a virgin. She mentions that she has already had intercourse with the son of the Director at summer camp, who had sexual encounters with several of her companions. HH cannot accept this, since he had tried to *create* Lolita. The fact that she has been initiated by another person, with a possible personal desire for him different to what he considers appropriate for her, is too hard to bear. He therefore tries to mold Lolita to his plan, in order to *make* her according to his desire: any different desire on her part would be severely punished. We should also mention that HH's manifest desire is an expression of an unwavering internal need: the drive increase he cannot process and the background of the underlying aphanisis.

HH and Lolita have repeated arguments because she refuses to accept the daily sexual routine imposed by him. At times they insult each other and eventually she threatens him with calling the police, so as to accuse her *father* of having raped her. She also complains of intense pain, unable to sit down because she feels her bowels destroyed.

In the middle of one of these fights, she asks him for money to call her mother at hospital. HH denies her the money but, after much insistence, he confesses that her mother is dead. At the next hotel, HH requests for two separate rooms but Lolita soon knocks on his door, entering the room, and they make love more gently. HH broods on his obtained satisfaction; since Lolita had nowhere to go, she was *forever* tied to him.

The interminable car trips continue around the United States, as HH tries to avoid suspicions. After the first shock of discovering Lolita was not a virgin, HH feels relieved and he ironically tells her that he is neither a psychopath nor a rapist but rather a *therapist*. He threatens her by saying that she must take care of the relationship because, if he went to jail, she would be confined to a reformatory for minors or an orphanage.

HH supposes that Lolita does not imagine that the endless trip is only a way of hiding the kind of relationship they have. Furthermore, he is jealous of an incipient and flourishing beauty in Lolita which he perceives is desired by all the men they come across. Even so, he makes an effort to give Lolita some freedom. He allows her to skate and tries to teach her to play tennis, although Lolita prefers to play with another girl. He also lets her bathe in a swimming pool, while he pretends to read a book. However, he does not take his eyes from her, remembering their last intercourse that morning. He recalls the pleasure of bringing her breakfast, denying it until she had obliged him. He also recalls the afternoon hours, as he sat ecstatically in an armchair with an indifferent Lolita on his lap.

But his active control of Lolita's activities represents not only fear but the terror of losing her, not only because of the resulting loneliness and abandonment but because of the profound concern that leads HH to the feeling of dying every time he moves away from her.

Intelligently, Nabokov leads the reader away from any eventual psychoanalytical interpretations. In his confession, which he imagines before a jury of psychoanalysts that will study his case, he maintains that the latter will be anxious to know whether he had intended to satisfy his frustrated desire for Annabel when he took Lolita to the seaside.

HH suggests getting married in Mexico, if they could only cross the border. He wishes to get Lolita pregnant so that she can conceive a new *nymphet* that will satisfy him in ten years' time, when she will no longer be able to do so. But HH begins to get tired and is running out of money, while Lolita becomes more and more radiant. Their disagreements, however, become so frequent that he decides to confine her to a boarding school for girls and ensures that he can watch her with binoculars from a rented room hired for that purpose. Shortly afterwards, he is summoned to the boarding school and is informed that Lolita is apparently not concerned about sexual issues; the authorities are worried about her sexual development. HH feels profoundly satisfied at this irony, imagining that his *education* has worked.

In the meantime, Lolita begins to take theatre classes, which she greatly enjoys. HH does not object, since the classes are supervised by the Institute. She also learns to play the piano but HH panics when he learns that she has been skipping classes without his knowledge. He therefore confronts her and tells her that she has to stop immediately, threatening her with boarding school if she does not change her behavior. He realizes that he is losing control over Lolita, since she finds different ways of deceiving him. Distraught, HH realizes that Lolita hates him and she reiterates that he had attempted to rape her when he was a tenant at her mother's house. Furthermore, Lolita accuses him of having murdered her mother, saying she would have sexual intercourse with whomever she wished and he would not be able to do anything about it.

At this point, Lolita escapes and HH finds her with great effort. She then tells him she has made a decision. They can renew their trip but from now on she will decide what route to take. HH accepts, although from then on he begins to feel persecuted. He cannot imagine what Lolita is trying to achieve, suspecting that she wants to free herself from him. In fact, she often leaves home without permission, returning some time later. He also observes her furtively talking with the employee of a gas station and, worst of all, the insistence with which a red car follows them, imagining that a private detective is monitoring their movements. Then, HH feels disillusioned and sorry for himself; how quickly the young *nymphets* forget everything while old lovers treasure each memory.

He resorts to physical violence, but Lolita continues with her schemes and the scenes of violence are followed by love and sex, lust and enjoyment, in an interminable continuum.

It seems as if HH's anxiety of death is increasing because he insists on his desire to cross the border and marry Lolita so that she can conceive a *nymphet*. This situation could consciously represent the fear of being left alone, without the sustenance Lolita represents, as well as the tension between drive increase and the background of the underlying aphanisis. This concern makes him accept the liberties Lolita violently tears from him: taking theatre and piano lessons, which HH pretends to control. In any event, HH perceives with despair that she is progressively escaping from him. Furthermore, his fear of aging is also evident, a dread that permeates the novel. This is manifested in his disillusionment with the young *nymphets*, who quickly forget their old lovers—as was stated above—who desperately cling to them.

The situation becomes more tense and HH imagines that all the cars that pass them on the highway are after them. Lolita, in turn, begins to feel sick and HH checks her into a hospital for two days, which separates him from her for the first time in two years. However, when he goes to pick her up, he is shocked to find out that Lolita has already left with an *uncle* the day before and, despite the scandal caused by his outrage, no further details are available. Finally, he realizes that he has to control himself, since it would be worse if he were detained by the police. He speculates that Lolita has fled with the detective that had been following them in one of the suspected cars.

Desperate, he returns to some of the hotels where they had stayed in order to check their registers for a clue that could help him find her captor, but this only makes him more confused and he decides to carry a gun with him, falling into a state of despair and pending doom.

Thus commences the end of the relationship, since the persecution could be understood as the emotional result of Lolita's attempt to find freedom. He experiences the separation with anxiety and when he takes her to the hospital he presupposes the end. He compares his separation as a door that opens violently to let in a merciless wind and black time. This irruption of time in his everyday life is what he has feared the most: chronological time dials aging and death, so different from the immortality he has been trying to find. He can only try to stifle his anguish crying for lone disaster.

During this period, he tries to seek other women, older than Lolita, although he admits the impossibility of *curing himself* of his pederosis, and he continues to haunt the places where they had shared important moments.

After a long time, he receives a letter from Lolita, telling him that she has married and is pregnant. She apologizes for not giving him her address because she imagines he must be upset with her; her husband, on the other hand, knows nothing of their relationship. She also asks him for money because she needs to go overseas, where her husband has a new job. HH, however, only thinks of murdering her husband, imagining that he must have been the one who followed them on the highway or one of the persons whom he had discovered chatting with her, when they were still together. Analyzing the letter's stamp, he cunningly manages to find out where they live, and drives in the car he has always used, which belonged to Clara. He finally arrives to their house feeling old and frail, foreshadowing the tragic end of a painful journey.

When Lolita opens the door, he sees the husband but absolves him from death, since the latter only knows HH is Lolita's father. However, in private, he demands to know who has been her kidnapper. After several attempts, Lolita confesses that her great love had been a playwright who had had serious problems due to his association with young girls. She confesses she had remained with him until he had suggested sexual group encounters, which she had dismissed as inappropriate for her. Nevertheless, he had followed her for several months, finally finding the opportunity to kidnap her when she was in hospital, with her complicity.

The attentive reader perceives then that the author had provided many clues of this relationship throughout the novel. Only at this point of Lolita's confession, however, these clues become clear. When she left the playwright, a friend of Lolita, who is now seventeen, introduced her to her present husband, with whom she is in love and expecting a child. HH forgives her for having been in love with another man and, notwithstanding her confession, he implores her to return with him. Lolita's refusal centers the plot in what we would like to demonstrate, since HH tells her that he feels old and frail. Once again, her presence attempts to mitigate the *experience* of aging, characteristic of the process of maturescence.

In his despair, HH highlights his concern regarding the passage of time, his aging and eventual death. He also emphasizes that they can be happy for the rest of their lives. Furthermore, the reference he makes to his old car, that she knows so well, could be a disguised reference of himself. He hastens to add that it would only take twenty-five steps to get inside the car. This could allude to the exact difference in age between them. Finally, he mentions death once again and begs her to die together. In one brief exchange of words, all these elements illustrate HH's dilemma of maturescence: he is unable to acknowledge his own aging, complicated by profound intra-psychic conflicts.

Lolita, however, vehemently refuses, even though HH gives her the money she had requested. HH then bursts into tears.

She then asks him where her *murdered* mother is buried. At this point, he remembers the death of his own mother and asks himself why he had never felt sorrow for that event. This provides another important nucleus of meaning because it is the only moment where HH cries; the only time he was able to connect with his affective life, emerging as a consequence of a drive increase confronted with the background of the underlying aphanisis. This moment enabled him to remember and integrate situations of his own life he had underestimated, such as the death of his own mother.

Lolita, in turn, apologizes for having let him down and thanks him for the money. From that moment onwards, HH does not stop until he has murdered the playwright, kidnapper and true lover of Lolita. The murder would be the natural culmination of the novel. What is at stake is not only the wish to *eliminate* the culprit of Lolita's liberation but also his desire for revenge, since the playwright had also disappointed her. Moreover we can consider that murdering him could represent the idea of killing a kind of double, who has led HH to a situation where there is no room for thought.

Finally, HH maintains that he has written his story in fifty-six days (the reader should note that Nabokov was fifty-six years old when he wrote the novel) and that he wishes that it should be published after both Lolita and himself have died. He apologizes for having killed the playwright, expressing that he had murdered him because he had to choose between him or his own self; he chose his victim because he wanted to live a few more months, so that Lolita and himself could live in the minds of later generations, the only immortality they could possibly share. Once again, the search for immortality evinces an unrestricted narcissism, characteristic of the ideal ego.

Arrested for murder, HH writes the book and dies of a coronary thrombosis a few days later, on November 16th, 1952. He does not know that Lolita had moved west; neither is he aware that she would die of childbirth days later, during Christmas, when she was giving birth to his daughter who was born dead, in a denouement reminiscent of classic Greek tragedy.

Perhaps HH's only comfort is to have died before *his* Lolita, closing his life history with slightly less sorrow than if it had been the other way around. His maturescence was profoundly influenced by his previous historic conflicts and his adult development was hampered by internal unsatisfied needs: devoid of the psychic resources for a working-through, the only course that enabled him to express his maturescent drive increase was an acting-out. Metaphorically, this author could say that HH achieved only one important thing: becoming part of the history of literature as one of the most fascinating characters ever created. This is no small feat and, possibly, the only way of remaining immortal, an issue that always concerned HH.

Returning to Nabokov, the following questions seem pertinent:

What could have been his motivation for writing the novel and creating a character like HH?

Why did he dedicate the novel to his wife Vera?

If his personal life could be studied, at what stages could we recognize HH in the life of the author?

These mysteries add unfathomable dimensions to *Lolita* but exceed the aims of this book; it is therefore left for specialists and readers.

Chapter 5

A reunion party

Mrs Dalloway (1925) by Virginia Woolf (1882–1941) also allows for an understanding of the maturescent working-through, although conscious contents—a consequence of the type of psychic functioning that prevails—may externally appear very different from those described in the novel *Lolita*—usually depicted as a midlife crisis. In *Mrs Dalloway*'s case, what can be inferred is a style of processing that could be characterized as a midlife transition. But the reader should not be confused; what this author is considering are two dissimilar types of psychic functioning and not the difference that could be found between men and women—regardless of the differences between climacterics in both sexes—since it would be possible to find women with the type of functioning shown by *Lolita*'s protagonist, Humbert Humbert, and men with the type of functioning displayed by *Mrs Dalloway*'s main character.

Mrs Dalloway takes place in only one day of the novel's protagonist, Clarissa Dalloway, who is about to have her fifty-second birthday after having overcome an apparent depressive state. Clarissa has decided to give a party at her London house. She feels rather anxious and worried, as if this social event were something quite important. She looks at herself in the mirror because she knows how dangerous it is to have spent her whole life waiting for only one thing: her party. She is determined to dazzle, awaken admiration, and be *the center of her own party*—with all the metaphoric sense that this last phrase can have in a psychoanalytic background.

The plot revolves around the flow of thoughts of the main characters, in the narrative style of stream of consciousness, characteristic of Woolf's writing. Clarissa is presented as a woman who has adapted to the social conventions of the time, becoming *Mrs* Dalloway. For many years she had stopped simply being Clarissa, even though she had tried to recover the Clarissa of her youth: a vital young girl full of dreams who had had an everlasting love and which continued to represent over the years a symbol of all she had lived.

But Clarissa not only believes that she has renounced to being herself; she also believes that everyone hoped she would get married and have children, becoming the wife of the prominent politician Richard Dalloway. She discovers, however, that her body no longer means anything to her, feeling almost invisible. This experience is characteristic of many maturescent women, as will be detailed in Chapter 6. Now that she has become fifty-two years old, Clarissa can hardly recognize her former self. She feels that she can no longer re-marry and particularly, that she can no longer have any more children. No longer the former Clarissa, it only remains for her to be *Mrs* Dalloway, *the wife of* Richard Dalloway.

Clarissa feels that she has betrayed herself; nevertheless, she has been partly happy. She cannot imagine a life different from the one she has led, but wishes to have lived another, more intense life. She perceives this conflict, this inner contradiction and feels the need to resolve it—a typical characteristic of maturescent conscious content.

For this reason, her interior monologue, where past and present intermingle, takes her back to her youth, rethinking and remembering her whole life history. At times she addresses herself as if she were young again and, at other times, as if she were the present Mrs Dalloway, often confronting one with the other.

As far as the present study is concerned, this author has considered the aspects of the plot that can be related to maturescence. Apart from Clarissa, other important characters in the novel (Peter, Richard, Sally, Hugh) experience similar dilemmas to that of the protagonist: the conflicts brought about by the phenomenon of maturescence. But before delving into the novel and its relationship to the topic, it's relevant to provide some basic information regarding the life of the author herself.

Virginia Woolf

Virginia Woolf (née Stephen), a British novelist and essayist, is considered one of the most prominent figures of modernism in the literary field as well as one of the greatest novelists of the 20th century. She was born in an environment where literature played an important part, since her father was an editor, critic and reputed biographer. As a result, many prominent authors used to visit Virginia's parental home. The literary classics of world literature, so ready at hand in the family library, gave Virginia a head start in the world of letters. Her mother, in turn, was very well connected, and she inherited from her the same bohemian tendencies as well as her beauty.

Virginia lived with her parents, her brothers and several other siblings that belonged to her parents' previous marriages, both widowed when they re-married. She described her father as a violent and selfish man, who used to shut himself for whole days feeling sorry for himself for not being recognized as a creative genius. Virginia had a difficult childhood, characterized especially by an apparently natural eccentricity and an uninterrupted series of small domestic accidents that led to mental imbalances that commenced since she was thirteen years old. At this time, in fact, her mother died unexpectedly and Virginia began to hear voices, a disturbance that grew worse when one of her half-sisters died two years later. Virginia often referred to her childhood both as a heaven and a hell.

The worst crisis, however, took place when Virginia's father died; at the time, she was twenty-two years old and had to be placed in a mental institution. By then, she not only heard voices but also refused to eat. Her hallucinations, for example, led her to perceive that the birds in her garden sang in Greek or that King Edward VII uttered all kinds of obscenities behind an enormous plant of azaleas. At this point, she attempted to commit suicide for the first time. Some biographers have also maintained that these early psychic disorders were caused by situations of sexual abuse which Virginia and her sister Vanessa suffered by two of her half-brothers when they were children. All these events were narrated in detail by Virginia herself in her diaries, where she also described her aversion to looking at herself in the mirror and her resistance to being photographed, despite her undoubted beauty. Her whole life was marked by these recurrent episodes which finally led her to take her own life. Moreover, her close bond with Vanessa, a conspicuous painter, was much more than a relationship between siblings and lasted throughout her lifetime— with all the ambivalent vicissitudes that characterize a fraternal bond. Vanessa could have functioned on many occasions as a referent of reality for Virginia.

A few years after the death of her father, Virginia, together with her siblings, decided to sell the paternal home. She then moved to the London neighborhood of Bloomsbury, where she experienced a kind of personal rebirth. Soon afterwards, she became acquainted with a group of young artists, forming the famous Bloomsbury group in 1910, which had an enormous influence in the aesthetic trends of the period. One member of the group was the prestigious intellectual Leonard Woolf, whom Virginia married in 1912. Five years later, they co-founded the famous publishing house the Hogarth Press, which enabled Virginia to publish her works without fear of censorship. The Hogarth Press is still one of the most important British publishing houses; some of its most renowned publications include the *Standard Edition of the Complete Psychological Works of Sigmund Freud*.

Some biographers maintain that the marriage was never consummated, since Virginia had always been attracted to women. Nevertheless, the bond between Virginia and Leonard was very strong. Her homosexual tendencies, on the other hand, were consummated when, in 1922, she began a relatively stable relationship with Vita Sackville-West, which lasted until her death. *Mrs Dalloway* was written in 1925, at a time when Virginia was involved with Vita. She was then forty-three years old. Critics consider this novel her first masterpiece, inaugurating her maturity as a writer. Virginia herself stated that the book marked a kind of watershed of her work.

Unfortunately, Virginia's mental health deteriorated, leading her to a profound depression. Some of the possible factors that contributed to her severe emotional collapse were the indifference of her literary critics, the onset of World War II and the consequent destruction of her London house. On March 28, 1941, at the age of fifty-nine, she filled her pockets with stones and drowned in the river near her home. Her body was found one month later and her husband buried her cremated remains in the garden of their home.

Virginia left Leonard a note where she wrote that she felt she was going mad. She had begun to hear voices again and was unable to work. The suicide note is undoubtedly a beautiful love letter where she confesses that no one had loved her as he had and that the few moments of happiness she had ever felt were due to his kindness. She did not think that two persons could have been happier than they had been. She could not find a better way out of her terrible situation than to take her own life, hoping that he would then be able to continue with his own work, unhindered by her illness.

Woolf was a prolific author. She wrote nine novels, more than seventy short stories, three unconventional novels which she termed *biographies*, in which she narrates the history of some well-known persons, including her own, more than ninety literary essays, a drama and travel books; her letters and diaries were published posthumously.

Mrs Dalloway was also made into a film (1997); and part of the plot was re-written by Michael Cunningham in the novel *The Hours* (1998), which had been the title originally suggested by Virginia Woolf for Mrs Dalloway. *The Hours* also has a film version (2002).

Mrs Dalloway

Until practically the end of the novel, the reader ignores the reason why Clarissa is giving a party, unaware whether it will commemorate something specific. It becomes clear, nonetheless, that for the hostess the celebration has a transcendental significance.

As has already been anticipated, Clarissa married an influential politician and enjoyed an excellent economic situation and position in society, surrounded by the London aristocracy of her day. She also had a daughter, Elizabeth. When she leaves home that morning in order to buy flowers for her party, she meets her old friend Hugh, who has also been invited to her *soiree*. The encounter takes her back to her youth and her boyfriend Peter, with whom she had broken up, refusing to marry him. Going to buy flowers could be equivalent to the steps a young girl takes when her first love appears. Clarissa, therefore, could be experiencing once again a kind of stepping out into the world after the illness that has afflicted her and kept her away from society for some time.

There is a poignant ambivalence about Clarissa. On the one hand, she feels very young but at the same time truly aged. She also experiences a certain remoteness, as if she were outside reality, at a distance that protects her from other people's threats. This self-assuredness is what enables her to enjoy her social ties. However, she is aware that being alive is also dangerous. These ambivalent feelings are key elements of her personality. Her continuous references to the passage of time are a human and painful mark. Furthermore, her personal and profound solitude is contrasted with her apparent social poise, making her a unique hostess, as her old flame Peter had predicted. She truly wishes to be committed to each instant of her life. At the same time, however, she seems afraid that living up to her inner wishes would place her emotionally at risk, since it would imply relinquishing the safety of remaining closed within herself.

The looking-glass is one of her favorite interlocutors, with whom she can converse about what she has lost. Looking into the mirror, she tells herself that words no longer mean anything. She has ceased to feel emotions, even though she can remember their previous intensity; for example, how she used to fix her hair in a state of sexual ecstasy when she was young. This description of a maturescent Clarissa resounds like the typical implosion of the body in front of the mirror, characteristic of the conscious maturescent comparison of one's present image with the memory of past ones, as it was referred in the chapter *Psychoanalysis of maturescence: the onset of middle age and beyond*.

Clarissa remembers one of the happiest moments of her life, when in the fullness of her youth she was about to meet her friend Sally Seton, with whom she was in love. She links these strong feelings with *Othello*'s lines: "If it were now to die 'twere now to be most happy" (Act 2, Scene 1). This emblematic link between love and death will recur later in the novel.

In her *dialogue* before the mirror, Clarissa begins to lament her lost vitality, as she recalls the plenitude of vital moments in her youth; the memory of her white dress serves as a symbol of her youth and beauty. Through these memories, Clarissa attempts to recuperate the vitality she feels is disappearing. It is worth remembering that these reminiscences are not the result of her illness but the other way around; her previous illness is a consequence of the need to process the maturescence she is so desperately trying to promote.

Looking at herself in the mirror reminds her of the moments she shared with her friend Sally, when they dreamt of abolishing private property, when her friend told her that she looked absolutely virginal. Although Clarissa had also strong feelings for Peter Walsh, she remembers her disappointment when the latter interrupts Clarissa and Sally's intimate moment, after Sally had kissed her on the mouth. Nevertheless, she admits she would have never dared to have a relationship of that nature.

The author also resorts to the theme of time by means of the omnipresent sound of London's Big Ben, a metaphor which permeates the novel. The clock's chimes serve as a backdrop that contrast human time—inevitably finite—with the eternal time that remains *alive* after death, a conscious characteristic of maturescence. A similar metaphor is employed in another novel by Woolf, *The Waves* (1931). A group of six friends describe their different ways of seeing the world, leading the reader to evoke the movement and sound of waves while the characters exchange viewpoints. The sound of the waves resound as an incessant echo throughout the novel in a similar way that Big Ben does throughout *Mrs Dalloway*: human life will pass, whereas the movement and sound of the waves, just like the sound of Big Ben, will remain in its incessant need to express an eternity that does not encompass human life.

As Clarissa is fixing the dress she will wear for her party, Peter Walsh unexpectedly irrupts into her drawing room, shaking them both emotionally, since they have not seen each other for many years. Peter feels that she has aged, attributing it perhaps to her previous illness. His immediate reaction, however, is to deny his own middle age, repeating to himself that he is not old. Clarissa, on the other hand, thinks he is looking well, and finds him just the same.

As Peter and Clarissa catch up with their news, she recalls their permanent quarrels and reconciliations. She also remembers how Peter expected everything from her, a commitment which she found stifling.

Even though they have not seen each other for a long time, their conversation demonstrates how their emotional bond has endured. Clarissa expresses her joy at seeing him and explains that she is mending the evening dress for the party she will give that evening. At the same time, she cannot help recalling old memories and asks herself why she had refused to marry him. She remembers how difficult this decision had been for her and finds Peter as charming as always. The permanent fluctuation between what she was in her youth and how she perceives herself now is another conscious evidence of the process of maturescence; a phenomenon that can promote these characteristic psychic changes and transformations.

Peter, who rashly married someone on his way to India, tells her that he is in love once again; he suspects that Clarissa might regard him as a failure, in comparison to how her own life has turned out. He explains that he has now fallen in love with a married woman, twenty-four years old, and has returned to London to obtain the necessary documents that will enable him to marry her. Unable to control his anguish, he bursts out crying, expressing his fear of another failure. Clarissa, in turn, attempts to console him, caressing him and kissing him on the cheek. At the same time, she cannot control a sudden longing: she wishes that he will take her away with him, almost as if he were about to set off on a journey. A question, then, is left unanswered: Peter asks her if she is happy but, just then, Clarissa's daughter Elizabeth appears. Once again, a sudden interruption occurs and Peter leaves in a hurry, while she runs after him to remind him of her party that evening.

The reader is also privy to Peter's thoughts. When he leaves Clarissa's house, he walks along Trafalgar Square thinking that it has been a long time since he felt so young. He commences to follow a young woman (following perhaps his lost youth?), still remembering Clarissa's pleading not to forget her party. He cannot help being surprised at the memories from his youth that come flooding to his mind as a consequence of having seen Clarissa once again. In his own way, Peter presents the same working-through maturescent style employed by Clarissa, despite their different personalities. However, although Clarissa considers that all is over for her (female menopause?), Peter cannot face up to the fact that he is now middle-aged, telling himself repeatedly that he is not old (male climacteric?).

Richard, on the other hand, also experiences similar memories when he learns that Peter Walsh is back in London. He recalls the moments shared with Peter and Clarissa when they were young. He asks himself what Peter's feelings would be now, remembering that Peter had been in love with Clarissa. After his luncheon engagement, therefore, he decides to buy some flowers for Clarissa, determined to express his feelings for her as soon as he arrives home, something which he never does.

The reader thus notes the tension brought about by the contrast of past with present, evincing the elaboration process Richard is undergoing, as well as certain contents of conscience that make evident the drive increase characteristic of maturescence. When he arrives home, Clarissa mentions that several guests will not be able to attend her party. Her husband asks her not to worry, concerned that the evening preparations could affect her health. But Clarissa is keen to make a success of her soirée; she feels particularly able to carry out these parties by creating a magical and fascinating atmosphere where everyone fees special, including herself.

Clarissa tells Richard that he is simpler than her and that he should have never married her. Richard then asks her what she would have done in that case, and she answers him that she would have married Peter Walsh. She tells him that Peter, in fact, visited her that morning, and that he was very much the same, an eternal youth, chronically immature, although still very lovable. Moreover, her elaboration of her maturescent processing goes much further. She asks herself if it would be enough to wake up every morning in order for life to have any meaning; if seeing the sun, walking in the park, meeting friends, seeing Peter once again, receiving her husband's roses were enough to make her happy. What more could one expect of life?

At this point, her concern regarding death appears. This author reminds the reader that the thesis of this book is that the conscious content of death would indicate the expression of the unconscious content of aphanisis—the underlying content of drive increase. Clarissa thinks that death seems incredible if contrasted to the plenitude of what she is experiencing at that moment; it seems absurd to her that everything should come to an end, after having enjoyed every instant of being alive, as she has done so far. Clarissa's transcendental theory allows her to cope with the anxiety of death. Despite her skepticism, she believes that the transitory aspect of life—the soma, in psychoanalytic terms—so fleeting, is ephemeral compared with the invisible part of life, which spreads in every direction. Moreover, that invisible part could somehow survive, and perhaps be recuperated somewhere, like a tormented soul, after death. This is the transaction she finds in order to evade, if only for a moment, the anguish of death: the promise of somehow recuperating life after death, expressing in this way that which seems inadmissible to human nature and which is intimately linked to the perception of aging during maturescence and ensuing middle age.

Clarissa writes Peter a thank-you letter, expressing her surprise and delight of having seen him once again. This leads Peter to an elaboration of some aspects of the passage of time and the perception of aging. He believes that passions always endure, maintaining their strength, but that life leads each person to add to their passions the supreme power of existence, which comes from experience. It is interesting here to compare Peter's ideas with the meaning of *experience* that will be presented in Chapter 6. Thus Peter balances the passions of his youth with what he is experiencing in middle age.

Peter also remembers his youth, when he had asked Clarissa to tell her the truth about her relationship with Richard, Clarissa told him that Richard made her feel secure and that she was not prepared to leave everything and go overseas with Peter. This evinces internal tensions between the known and the unknown, endogamy and exogamy, for example. Peter then tells her that Richard would keep her imprisoned in a perfect jail, full of flowers and elegant furniture, even though she thought Richard would leave her with breathing space, a space that Peter himself did not give her. It was then that Clarissa told him their relationship was over, running away as if she were escaping from herself. Despite all these memories, however, Peter decides to attend Clarissa's party.

When the reception commences, Clarissa is quite nervous, fearing that her party will be a failure, thus demonstrating how much of her own self is at stake. Nevertheless, she is happy to see that Peter has come. The latter greets Richard, expressing how long it has been since they have seen each other. Clarissa is afraid that Peter will get bored, since he hardly knows anyone; she is also afraid that he will criticize her party. Peter, in turn, observes her from a distance with a carefree and mischievous attitude, as she receives her aristocratic guests, noticing her preoccupation for the evening's success.

Another surprise for Clarissa is the sudden appearance of Sally Suton, now Lady Rosseter, who attends the party. She has come uninvited, since she happens to be in town with her husband. Delighted to see them, Clarissa tells her two old friends that she will talk to them later in the evening.

Using the narrative technique of stream of consciousness, the author allows the reader to penetrate into the thoughts of all the main characters, letting them perceive the tension each one experiences, as well as their own maturescent working-through, as they compare their current lives with their expectations when young: the past has returned with the identities of adult life. Even though the novel is centered around Clarissa; Peter, Richard and Sally come physically together after many years, undergoing similar internal processes of elaboration.

With the party well under way, Clarissa wonders around the different rooms and cannot help reflecting on life and death; she considers the importance and potentiality the gift of life has, given by parents when a child is born—a life that has to be lived to the full until the end—; moreover, she feels intimidated when she perceives this so clearly. In a way, she confuses the conscience of finitude with the experience of plenitude. This is characteristic of maturescence and ensuing middle age in light of the elaboration of individual's life course. At times, she sees her guests as actors, lit up by spotlights that will soon afterwards disappear to enable other guests to play their part, while she remains conscious of the whole scene. Although she realizes that nothing lasts for too long, she also feels immensely happy, perhaps happier than she has ever felt. However, she also asks herself whether, over the course of so many years beside Richard, often feeling dull and disappointed, she has not lost an essential part of herself.

As Richard proudly dances with his daughter, Sally and Peter discuss Clarissa's marriage. Perhaps she had needed someone who regarded life as a simple affair. Peter tells her that Clarissa had broken his heart and that such intense feelings could only be experienced once. Clarissa had a purity, a charm and a generosity that were unique. Although he is not quite sure what his present feelings are, he knows that his previous love for Clarissa has remained with him up to now, giving a unique sense to his life. The reader also perceives that something similar has happened to Clarissa. Both Peter and Clarissa are promoting maturescent working-through processes that will allow them to carry on with their lives. This is also made evident when Peter maintains that the intense feelings of youth do not allow a person to see people as they are, only becoming possible when one is older. He considers that now that he is fifty-three he can see, understand and preserve the capacity to feel. He coincides, therefore, with Sally who also admits a greater depth and passion with the years, to which Peter suggests adding one's experience.

The ability of Virginia Woolf to lead the reader into the stream of consciousness of each character is remarkable. She manages to convey the fact that they are all tryng to elaborate the emotional experiences of their youth, which is paradigmatic of the processes that normally occur in maturescence and ensuing middle age.

The novel ends when Peter begins to feel very anxious as he awaits Clarissa's return. He experiences a mixture of ecstasy and terror, an incredible excitement, until he realizes that it is due to Clarissa herself, who has finally appeared.

This author would like to conclude by referring to one of the recurring symbols of the novel: flowers. The novel commences with Clarissa going out to buy flowers for her party. She remembers the floral arrangements her girlfriend Sally used to make when she came to visit her at her family home: one of Clarissa's most intense moments was when she was going to meet Sally. Her husband Richard also brings her flowers on the day of the party, which she places on the mantelpiece. Finally, Elizabeth, Richard and Vanessa's young daughter, is often compared to flowers. This symbolic resource operates as a powerful organizer of the main characters and the plot in general; it could represent the *somatic fertility* that clouds Clarissa, as well as the rest of the maturescent characters, even if what Clarissa and the others are searching for is a *creative fertility* through the naturalness, freshness and intensity that a flower represents. Both kinds of fertility are present and characterize the maturescent process.

At the same time, flowers, cut in order to become ornamental objects, possess an ephemeral quality similar to human life, only surviving for a certain while. Therefore, the reader could consider whether Clarissa would not be expressing by means of flowers a concern for her own life as having been torn and condemned to the brief and traumatic interlude life offers; something quite opposite to achieving the full development implicit in a life without these vicissitudes, a project that would seem possible after her maturescent working-through. This torn life could represent her decision when young to abandon Peter; however it returns during the maturescent processing with a different psychic content.

Similarly, the party brings together Clarissa, Richard, Peter and Sally, who cannot help reviving intense memories of their youth. These memories force them to consider their current situation and what they have actually done with their lives. This is another important aspect of maturescence and ensuing middle age: coming into terms and new balance and tension between ideal ego and ego ideal.

We could consider then that Clarissa attempts to elaborate the emotional states that are usually activated as questions during maturescence and ensuing middle age. As expected, these emotional states represent situations that often cannot be clearly resolved. They imply instead the irruption of enigmas which each person must sustain, accepting an uncertain destiny for each of these questions. The experience of uncertainty, therefore, occupies a central role in each maturescent individual. For all these reasons, Clarissa Dalloway's life serves as a paradigmatic example of the effort to understand a midlife transition as a path for a maturescent working-through.

Chapter 6

Different understandings of maturescence

Let us now consider both an indirect and a direct understanding of maturescence. An *indirect understanding of maturescence* refers to the confusion between manifest and latent contents of psychic processes and individual experiences. It is easy to find papers about losses during midlife—more specifically during middle age; for example, the loss of parents, the so called empty nest syndrome (when children leave the parental home), the loss of a youthful body, the loss of a contemporary (a "double," originally doomed to immortality), and many more, assuming they are universals. But these situations may also happen at different moments during the life cycle. Furthermore, they involve external and manifest evidences, only implying the conscious way the patient has to tell us what is *happening* and *experiencing* with the best words he can find. Nevertheless, as analysts, we must *translate* these events into an interpretation referred to the true latent content which is different from what the patient says.

Analyzing it from the logic of dreams, we rely on manifest dream content just as a hint, a faint light that guides us towards true latent dream thoughts, but we do not assign truth value to the manifest content. When a patient is speaking about his sorrow because his children aren't living with him anymore, we can conceive of a vertex from which he is referring to that sorrow. However, that situation is not directly related to his maturescence because that is only the manifest or indirect evidence.

The *direct understanding of maturescence*, on the other hand, considers what is happening with the psychic expression of somatic phenomena related to climacterics in men and women and the possibility of working-through an outcome for *the revolt against biology*—let's say: maturescence. This does not mean, however, that reproduction is the key; on the contrary, maturescence is a universal phenomenon that goes far beyond reproduction itself; it is linked to a somatic process rooted in nature and expressed in the body.

An individual may have had several children and will necessarily live the same process which will be noticed as well because it is not related to whether or not he has had children but with the quantity of inner resources to work-through this situation, rooted in the *revolt against biology* (Bergler, 1954)—

and perhaps confronted with the background of the underlying aphanisis (Jones, 1927) later on as well—because maturescence is mostly the psychic outcome of the somatic decrease (men) or the somatic losing (women) of the possibility of the reproductive function.

Perhaps these ideas may be regarded as fundamentally biological, leaving psychoanalytic thinking in the background. However, it is quite the contrary because it is impossible to consider psychoanalysis without the biological ground that upholds it. There is no psychic life without the life of matter. Undoubtedly, there is a great resistance in the understanding of these aspects but as analysts we must go beyond what is understood as common sense. These resistances confuse what *may* happen during middle age with *the specific and determining issues* of the maturescent phenomenon which is universal.

This author does not agree with the concept of the empty nest syndrome or the illness, aging or death of one's own parents as universal middle age features. In fact, there are people who have not had children and will also experience this maturescent working-through process with their resources. There are also many people who have lost their parents long before they reached their fifties; nevertheless, they will go through the same process. Even those who have had eighty or ninety year old healthy parents will undergo the same maturescent process.

Undoubtedly there is a deep resistance to an authentic understanding of what unites human beings to their biological life, as if we continued to believe we had a soul split from our body, a soul that lives within a body, instead of thinking that we are a soma with a psychic life that has a relative autonomy, in many cases a marvelous autonomy; although in others this autonomy may be so frightening as to begin wars against other human beings—*war* as a specifically human event.

A truly specific metapsychology of maturescence and ensuing middle age can be acknowledged only after we take into account the enormous *revolt against biology* that features maturescent working-through processing. And this *revolt against biology* is a universal due to drive increase. Only after this acknowledgement can we consider ideals, identifications, the renewal of the Oedipal conflict, narcissism and inter and intra generational vicissitudes.

From this vertex, we can consider the full metapsychology of psychoanalysis but rooted in the somatic substrate that connects us with our species and with biology. Only from this acknowledgement can we think of the best human realizations, the fabulous human conquests of imagination, fantasy, illusion, hope, the human achievements of arts, architecture, engineering, medicine, psychoanalysis itself, achievements in anthropology and history; as well as the human tragedies to which we are accustomed to, in a different way and differently from what happens with the rest of the living species, which do not suffer from the same inter-species destinies that human beings experience.

In the beautiful documentary *The Midlife Project* (2013), the American director Lori Petchers interviews women regarding menopause in order to seek their opinions. The video begins with a woman who says that as soon as she ceased to be fertile, she felt that she was treated as if she were invisible.

The great challenge of maturescence is transforming reproductive invisibility into psychic work—*the revolt against biology*—that could allow us to find a proper and individual answer, not a previous one taken from a book, a supposed wise man or a religious precept, but simply an individual answer allowing us to decide what to do with this pretended invisibility alluded to in the documentary. Invisibility is related to aphanisis—the hidden side of drive increase—the fear of the disappearance of one's own sexual desire and the concomitant fear of not being desired by others, which happens to both men and women.

Deviants of thought and the comprehension of maturescence

By *deviants of thought* this author means the psychic resources that force humans to deny their belonging to nature. They function as distracting elements that make a *de-centering* of subjectivity with respect to nature possible. Paradoxically, they were the elements that founded and made possible psychic life—the representation of instinct, in Freudian terms. These *deviants of thought* lead to a vision in inverted perspective of the authentic maturescent processes, since the background—natural somatic source of everything—disappears and humans can only notice the foreground, similarly to Plato's metaphor of the cavern, which served to explain human knowledge, as was suggested earlier. Briefly: the peril of an indirect understanding of maturescence.

This author could sustain that the *deviants of thought* exist at any moment during the life cycle, not only during maturescence. However, the proposal implies considering their specific transcendence in those moments when the somatic factor comes first. The two *princeps* moments, therefore, would be adolescence and maturescence, according to this theory. At those moments, the *deviants of thought* urge the denial of belonging of *human nature* vis-à-vis *biological nature*—the latter being the only *nature* worth considering, since the adjective biological would be redundant. For this reason, this vertex suggests that these *deviants of thought* lead to an indirect understanding of maturescence.

Five *intruders of thought* will be described below:

1. The narcissistic blows
2. Experience as (possible) resistance
3. Euphemisms
4. Common sense
5. Common places

Narcissist *de-centering* and *re-centering* by means of narcissistic blows

Understanding maturescence implies working on a human *re-centering* that leads to deposing the *de-centered* narcissist perspective in order to prioritize the *natural* perspective: the acknowledgment that human beings are part of nature. This author could even venture to affirm that human beings are not only part of nature but, simply, nature. How could narcissism be considered from a *de-centered* perspective? It is interesting to consider narcissism as a de-centered functioning, since—psychologically speaking—it would imply a priori a centering in the person himself. However, from the perspective of the natural processes of this theorization, narcissism is a *de-centered* functioning.

The existence of important psychic resistances at the service of a narcissistic positioning operate against this evidence, forcing the de-centering of reality from human nature. These resistances may be considered as *deviants of thought* because they promote the illusion of the possibility of *de-centering* the individual from nature.

When Freud (1917a) held that scientific research promoted three severe narcissistic blows for humanity: cosmological, biological and psychological, he was sustaining how narcissism influences the *de-centering* already alluded to; something difficult to *re-center*: an anthropocentric perspective. The self-sufficiency, the arrogance, the disdain, etc. vis-à-vis the rest of the natural species, are reactions that make evident the defenses that human beings can or try to implement in order to deny being part of nature.

Even if way before Copernicus, the idea that the Earth was smaller than the sun and went around it had already been exposed, it was with Copernicus that human narcissism experienced the first cosmological affront.

The biological affront appears with Darwin's theories, his precursors and collaborators. Freud (1917a) sustains:

> Man is not a being different from animals or superior to them; he himself is of animal descent, being more closely related to some species and more distantly to others. The acquisitions he has subsequently made have not succeeded in effacing the evidences, both in his physical structure and in his mental dispositions, of his parity with them.
>
> [p. 141]

The tenet of the three affronts is reconfirmed by Freud when he maintains that the third affront, according to him, the most painful, is the psychological one because with the discovery of unconscious processes brought about by psychoanalysis:

> The ego is not master in its own house.
>
> [p. 143]

What leads human beings to maintain this denial of reality as a *de-centering*?

Perhaps the answer could be that Freud proposed these three affronts of humanity's narcissism as a denial recourse, which becomes evident with the results of scientific research. Going deeper, however, they imply a progressive discovery of the de-centering that humanity, and each individual in particular, implemented in order to sustain psychic life: a kind of structuring affront of psychic life. More important than the narcissistic wounds, therefore, would be to consider the reasons why this denial was necessary.

This author could also interpolate here an idea that may seem contrary to the Freudian claim when he considers that this third affront could stem from the second (the biological one), and would be much more powerful than the others. The biological affront pretends to confront with an unrestricted narcissism, which already implies a form of psychic existence—in the same way that the cosmological affront implies a form of psychic existence. From this perspective, the psychological affront would be present in the cosmological and biological affronts from the beginning of human existence.

Perhaps it could be sustained that psychoanalysis was able to discover the violence implied by the essential *de-centering* arising from cosmological and especially, biological affronts, almost as if it had served as the instrument that made the understanding of the nature of these affronts possible; it is surprising that the word *nature* seems over-determined by two facets. This author could therefore suggest at this stage a psychological affront, as long as we admit that it traverses the other two, being implicit in both.

Experience as (possible) resistance

One of the *deviants of thought* that foster an indirect comprehension of maturescence is the idea that increased *experience* (or so-called accumulated experience) is sufficient to consider that some of the specific qualities attributed to the maturescent process can start to appear spontaneously.

The reader may find here two different meanings and senses for the word *experience*: a *real* one and a *defensive* one.

Thus conceived, life experience would seem to be a maceration process whereby an internal disposition, uniform and with its own identity, begins to take shape. However, this affirmation is contradicted by psychoanalytic clinical work because some individuals are able to muster experience very easily, while for others it is impossible—compulsion to repeat leads the latter to the impossibility of learning from experience, as Bion (1962) said. There is evidence that a multiplicity of individual destinies exists—impossible of being summarized in any series—that can only be understood from an individual internal perspective.

The concept of experience, however, must be used carefully because what experience really means can be confused with the simple passage of time, thus promoting a kind of false comprehension or the evidence of a new psychic resistance similar to a *deviant of thought.*

Perhaps it might be clarified that *authentic experience* cannot be provided only by years: it would need something else, a way of *living the actual moment,* which is not universal either. Possibly, everyone who goes through maturescence can affirm that they have a certain accumulated experience, and they may speak from that place. Nevertheless, what is expressed individually is not sufficient for it to be valued as an authentic experience. Who could maintain the contrary about himself? The question would be, on the one hand, how and when an (authentic) experience is sufficient to sustain the idea of the acquisition of characteristics attributed to having worked-through maturescence; and, on the other, when is the word *experience* used as resistance.

There's something else that could be added to the passing of years; a differential plus so that we could refer to experience, or more specifically to the so-called accumulated experience. That extra plus, which is not always present, is related to a kind of search, a purpose—perhaps an overcoming purpose—that goes further than simply wishing to find pleasure at all times, that can emphasize the *living the actual moment.*

What word could provide an adequate definition to account for *experience?*

Perhaps the idea that the transition from the past (accumulated experience) to the continuous present (living the actual moment) can provide a certain clarity. It is very different to refer to accumulated experience—that which has already been lived—than to allude to *the experience that is being accumulated at the present moment.* This continuous present may provide the difference that would allow us to emphasize what can be referred to as experience, since not all experience is authentic; least of all, accumulated experience, even in the absence of notorious psychopathologies.

Individuals could also regard experience from a defensive aspect. If faced with an uncertain situation at a certain point in an individual's life, they resort to previous experience, or the so-called accumulated experience, previous experience, or life experience. Thus, individuals will be losing the immense opportunity of confronting the uncertainty which that unique moment of his life is presenting. And here a great difference occurs, which could be termed as a qualitative difference. There will be those who, in specific situations, feel themselves summoned to this retroactive vision—a way of appealing to previous experience with the risk of *avoiding* the present experience. On the other hand, there will be those who will prefer to confront the unknown, not allowing any shadow of the past to remove them from that moment. Two different destinies are opened here: avoidance and confrontation, similar to the *de-centering* and *re-centering* already alluded to.

To give a simple example, this would be similar to the habit of taking photographs when travelling or at certain events. Photography is an extraordinary resource which allows us to capture reality in two dimensions, withdrawing it from time. Undoubtedly, if we considered it in this way, a philosophical treaty could be elaborated—the shifting of reality to different dimensions that would contain it, for example, with a relative accuracy of the image. However, it would be a philosophical treatise with a certain experience, since the individual who takes the photo is trying to retain something forever—the photograph as an illusion that captures a moment-of-eternity or for-eternity. But—following Barthes (1980)—if "Photography is a certificate of presence" [p. 134], "Photography does not (forcefully) say what is no more but merely and undoubtedly what has been" [p. 132], because "in Photography, the immobilization of time only occurs in an excessive way, monstrous: time is stuck" [p. 140].

At the precise moment the individual takes the photograph, he remains outside the experience of living that moment—as stuck as time in photography, following Barthes—, hiding from that reality with the excuse of preserving it forever. This constitutes a strange paradox; instead of living that moment, he is evading the experience he is trying to preserve with the excuse of perpetuating it because of its transcendence, beauty, interest, etc., leading him to an empty experience. If this individual would comment his trip to a third person, he would probably talk about what he experienced, but was it really an *authentic* experience, an accumulated one, or should we find some other word that could describe what he lived? So, what can really determine the authenticity of accumulated experience? It is evident that the interpolation regarding the photographic question is valid: in the example of the travel photograph—although the example should not be taken as an absolute.

Considering experience with another example, we can find a similar difference to the one provided previously regarding photography by comparing it to the experience of watching a film. A movie watched at home is never the same as seeing the same movie at the cinema. Has the reader ever asked himself why the remembrance of a movie seen at the cinema is much more intense? The home experience implies the supposed advantage of being able to press *Pause* at will, or *Playback*, if the spectator wishes to revise some aspect of the film, or simply stopping it to prepare something to eat or drink and renewing the screening later. But these advantages collapse when we try to internally register the authentic experience of watching a film at the movie theater. Firstly, we must be punctual, try not to lose any details, and we certainly cannot reproduce again certain parts of the film. All these disadvantages, however, give us the benefit of having a truly authentic experience *at the movies'*, in contrast with the comfort of seeing it at home. The vital force of remembering the film seen at movie theater is always more intense. The two remembrances are different and this is similar to the difference between the experience of a tourist enjoying his trip or a tourist who meticulously registers photos of the trip. In the case of the movie theater, not being able to manipulate or detail chronological time adds value to the experience whereas seeing the film at home produces the opposite effect.

This author states that *confrontation* with the present moment with the pretense of perpetuating it makes *true experience* disappear, whereas in the allusion to the *life experience* as something that can be capitalized in moments of the life cycle that demand confronting specific uncertainties, an equivalent phenomenon could take place: *confrontation* with the present moment also disappears, with the pretense of having the resources to capitalize it better, resulting in the triumph of *avoidance*. It sounds almost identical. Therefore, *true experience* is something else.

The *Oxford English Reference Dictionary* defines *experience* as:

> —*n.* 1 actual observation of or practical acquaintance with facts or events.
> 2 knowledge or skill resulting from this. 3 an event regarded as affecting one (*an unpleasant experience*). b the fact or process of being so affected (*learned by experience*).
> —*v.tr.* 1 have experience of; undergo. 1 feel or be affected by (an emotion etc.).

On the other hand, *Webster's New Universal Unabridged Dictionary* defines *experience* as:

> —*n.* 1 a particular instance of personally encountering or undergoing something: *My encounter with the bear in the woods was a frightening experience.* 2. the process or fact of personally observing, encountering or undergoing something: *business experience.* 3. the observing, encountering, or undergoing of things generally as they occur in the course of time: *to learn from experience; the range of human experience.* 4. knowledge or practical wisdom gained from what one has observed, encountered or undergone: *a man of experience.* 5. *Philos.* the totality of the cognitions given by perception; all that is perceived, understood, and remembered.
> —*v.t.* 6. To have experience of; meet with; undergo; feel: *to experience nausea.* 7. to learn by experience.

Please note that in these definitions, the first meaning in both dictionaries is directly linked to the proposal presented here:

> —*n.* 1 actual observation of or practical acquaintance with facts or events. (OERD)
> —*n.* 1 a particular instance of personally encountering or undergoing something. (WNUD)

Only the meanings that follow consider what this author has termed a mode of understanding *experience* as resistance, something which directly leads to an indirect understanding of maturescence.

Euphemisms: sex and death

Common language and popular expressions also may work as expressions of the *deviants of thought*. One of these deviants are euphemisms. The *Dictionary of Euphemisms and Other Double-talk* (Rawson, 1995), an unbelievable book with hundreds of entries with euphemisms and double-talk with full and deep explanations, has its place here. Everybody can confirm with this dictionary the reality of psychoanalytical truths: euphemisms and double-talk have to do mostly with sex and death! There are no contents so frequently mentioned as sex and death in the different entries of this Dictionary.

It could be argued against these statements that psychoanalysis discovered that sex and death are the most important topics to be considered—that this is nothing new—but perhaps the reader could also consider these ideas as two of the core concepts of *maturescence*, as this theorization is attempting to demonstrate.

The author defines euphemisms as:

"Mild, agreeable or roundabout words used in place of coarse, painful, or offensive ones." The term comes from the Greek *eu*, meaning "well" or "sounding good," and *pheme*, "speech" … Yet euphemisms have very serious implications. They conceal the things we fear most—death, the dead, the supernatural. They cover up the facts of life—of sex, reproduction and excretion—which inevitably remind even the most refined people that they are made of clay, or worse … As such, they are outward and visible signs of our inward anxieties, conflicts, fears, and shames"

(Rawson, 1995) [p. 1]

Euphemisms and double-talk could be considered *deviants of thought* because they try to express (indirectly) but can't express (directly) what they mean with the same word. The dictionary, in fact, cannot have a version in reverse. If it were possible, there would be very few entries, all of them related to sexual content—especially the genitals (male and female sex organs: penis and vagina, reproduction of the human species and so on)—and death content —especially death (with all its variations: illness, convalescence, death itself, the so called afterlife, cemeteries, etc.).

The printed version with all the euphemisms and double-talk—as was already stated—has hundreds of entries and all of them could be considered as always being renewed because language is a *living thing* and these transformations are permanently updated, turned into the aftermaths that show unconscious hints revealing omnipresent and *eternal* unconscious contents: sex and death.

Let's consider several examples (all page numbers refer to Rawson, 1995). Related to **sex**:

- **organ**: women have internal organs but as a rule only men have external, euphemistic *organs*, i.e., the penis (aka the *male generative organ* or the *reproductive organ*), the testicles (or *male organs*), and the collective *organs or generation* (p. 301);

- **commerce**: a mercantile metaphor for sex—what *The Oxford English Dictionary* primly defines as "intercourse of the sexes: *esp*. in the bad sense" (p. 86);
- **parts**: sexual parts (p. 309);
- **romance**: love outside marriage or, more specifically, sex (with or without marriage) (p. 361);
- **tool**: the penis (p. 425);
- **panties**: women's underpants; the diminutive minimizes the sexual associations by casting the adult wearers in the roles of children or little girls (p. 306);
- **menstruation** has a lot of euphemisms, sometimes conveying the idea of illness or inconvenience, also called "the red color," "periodicity," "visit," "sexual unavailability," etc. (p. 274).

Related to **death**:

- **deceased**: dead, the dead person. This is probably the most popular way of not saying "dead" (p. 112);
- **pass away**: to die; an old euphemism (p. 309) [also "depart," "loss," etc.];
- **loved one, the**: dead person, the (p. c261);
- **sunset years**: old age (p. 407);
- **space**: a grave site (p. 395);
- **slumber cot/robe/room**: the "slumber" is very deep, for this is the sleep of the dead. A **slumber cot** is a coffin, a **slumber robe** is a shroud, and a **slumber room** is a lying-out room in a funeral room (p. 388).

Interestingly, and in the line of this book's theorization, could be found some euphemisms that bring together both **sex and death**:

- **die**: to experience sexual orgasm; a predecessor of the modern "come" (p. 123);
- **off**: to kill or to "screw," the commingling of death and sex in a single word being fairly standard practice (p. 299).

Where does this need to transform a proper word come from? Why is it necessary to change a word in order to speak specifically about sex and death? Why are these *deviants of thought* necessary? What might the reader think?

For sure, a contradiction may be found in these statements because this author —following Freud (1915b) [p. 289], (1923b) [p. 58]—already spoke about the unconscious impossibility of conceiving the idea of death. Again, sex and death are words that depict unconscious feelings (latent content) and euphemisms and double-talk are words that try to show unconscious reality—but without anxiety (manifest content). The power of the two moratoria this author proposes for the human life cycle are the answer to the need for euphemisms, a concept that confirms all psychoanalytic statements.

Euphemisms, then, especially those related to aging as deviants of thought, are also essential in order to understand working-through processes during maturescence, not only as a way of referring to maturescence itself, but also by providing psychoanalysts with a further tool when a maturescent patient refers to his life and interests. Moreover, euphemisms are a privileged way of expression when deep somatic processes are at work during maturescence and the individual tries to find the proper word to express his feelings.

Common sense and the effort to find one's own sense

The *Oxford English Reference Dictionary* defines *common sense* as one of the meanings of the word *common*: "sound practical sense, esp. in everyday matters," whereas the *Webster's New Universal Unabridged Dictionary* has its own meaning: "sound practical judgement that is independent of specialized knowledge, training, or the like; normal native intelligence."

Both definitions allude to what is being suggested, running the risk of thought approaching that median that usually blocks clear proposals—the reader must not forget the photograph metaphor—which allow us to go beyond common thought, transcending that lazy mediocrity that evinces creative numbness. Once again: the need to confront or avoid uncertainty and paradox.

One of the keys could be found in the word *logic*, since that which seems *logical* usually lacks the essential radiance needed to promote by means of thought those questions that can function as new starting points, instead of the time-worn tranquilizers that paralyze it. In other words, common sense functions as a factor that dulls our reasoning by providing an answer that closes it down—a *deviant of thought*—instead of offering an opening that could lead to new challenges.

Generally, when someone refers to common sense, the avoidance of a process of authentic thought is made evident. It functions as a kind of false *democratization* which presupposes that everyone will coincide with what is being affirmed because it is a truth that well-meaning people accept a priori without question.

Unfortunately, however, this is where the error commences because the so-called common sense, once it is set in motion, promotes a paralysis of thought which is almost impossible to transgress, obstructing the road towards new horizons: an apparently threatening alternative, but full of enthusiasm nevertheless. An example can be provided with what was previously discussed regarding experience. From the point of view of common sense, *life experience* is obtained by the simple passage of years, giving it thus a universal character. We maintain, however, that *authentic* experience is something quite different.

Common sense, in other words, provides the false warmth of that which is familiar. It promotes a false identification with the subject, leading him to believe that there are previous assumptions that must be shared by all. These universal truths, which cannot be questioned because they have already been established, encompass those this author has previously considered when he dealt with experience and euphemisms: truths that belie the urgency to deny that, whether we like it or not, we are akin to nature; what sex and death confirmed with the discovery of psychoanalysis.

The use of the so-called common sense ends up functioning as a suffocating mechanism that dulls thought. In the case of a relationship with another speaker, it aims at obtaining an identification with the other person, hoping to be accepted since, after all, they both share a reassuring common vision. We could almost regard this phenomenon as an agreement where both parties establish a common comfort zone to maintain the *status quo*. Psychoanalysis employs the term *bastion* or *bulwark* (Baranger, 1961): that *special thing* which cannot be discussed either by the patient and the analyst or by the analyst and the patient.

We should note that the *common place* (*cliché*) which alludes that "common sense is the least common of all the senses" is not mentioned. This expression reinforces the power of closure that this *deviant of thought* has. In fact, in supposedly valuing common sense, what it really provokes is a reinforcement of the supposed value of *common sense*, as it often occurs with them, thus linking meanings.

Be this as it may, a strong philosophic tradition exists regarding common sense which usually defines it as the sum total of all the original principles that can be found in normal minds, proposing it as a series of universal convictions of humanity. These would include beliefs and propositions emanating from society as a whole, even though it would not seem to admit questionings.

The same philosophic tradition—with some (falsely) religious interferences—suggest that "common sense" implies a form of knowledge, differentiating degrees that would range from *common sense*, science, philosophy ... and faith.

Descartes' definition is quite surprising, because he considers common sense as the most fairly distributed thing in the world, for each one thinks he is so well-endowed with it that even those who are hardest to satisfy in all other matters are not in the habit of desiring more of it than they already have. In other words, Descartes sustains that common sense is the ability to distinguish what is true from what is false—the reality of fantasy, in the context of the present analysis. Moreover, common sense is a reaction in light of those actions that are not premeditated and which depend on chance.

It is worth considering these ideas because the importance and centrality of uncertainty was already discussed in Chapter 2, including its unpredictability, during maturescence. This would seem to be related with what is not premeditated and with chance, according to the Cartesian premises.

Those who are capable of confronting uncertainty, with all its characteristics, will be in a position to promote their *own sense* of individual thought. This is not only useful from the perspective of maturescence but is also in tandem with the overcoming purpose implicit to transcend *common sense* and achieve one's *own individual sense*.

A good example of this passage is provided by the British lexicographer Samuel Johnson (1709–1784), author of the first dictionary of the English language, since he seems like the archetype of common sense, his own voice always resounding in his thought, often paradoxically. Let us consider some examples:

> My congratulations to you, sir. Your manuscript is both good and original; but the part that is good is not original, and the part that is original is not good.
>
> I never desire to converse with a man who has written more than he has read.
>
> The chains of habit are too weak to be felt until they are too strong to be broken.
>
> That we must all die, we always knew; I wish I had remembered it sooner.
>
> (Johnson, 2009, p. 126)

The *common places* and the closure

Common sense reveals itself as a close relation of *common place*; they share a second degree kinship. Furthermore, common sense seems to perform functions equivalent to closure or blockage. Some examples of colloquial speech share this mixed nature between *common sense* and *common place*; for example, in expressions that refer to aging:

1. "To grow old graciously"
2. "A woman of certain age"

The first expression also functions as a euphemism because it pretends to smooth over the reality of aging with all that the latter entails, whereas the second saying, in its indetermination regarding age, tries to achieve the same objective.

This original meaning of *common place* is derived by extension to the vulgar denotation of something intranscendental which is used to define a phenomenon that always occurs in the same manner. In all cases they reveal a lack of originality and linguistic resources.

Most proverbs function as common places, since they are repeated almost without thinking. Sancho Panza, Don Quixote's squire and companion, provides a great example of the use of these common places or sanchismos; he constantly refers to sayings, so worn and repeated that they have become meaningless. In his innocence, he maintains: "And I have got nothing else, nor any other stock in trade except proverbs and more proverbs." (Part II, Chapter XLIII). What he is saying to Don Quixote is not to expect any true thoughts from him because he only has proverbs to offer.

Here are some examples, among the hundreds Sancho utters, which illustrate their current validity, considering the four centuries that have elapsed since Cervantes first published this masterpiece of world literature:

"There's remedy for everything except death." (Part II, Chapter X)
"Only make yourself honey and the flies will suck you." (Part II, Chapter XLIII)
"The dead woman was frightened at the one with her throat cut." (Part II, Chapter XLIII)
"The fool knows more in his own house than the wise man in another's." (Part II, Chapter XLIII)
"A man may come for wool and go back shorn." (Part II, Chapter XIV)

Don Quixote himself often complains of Sancho's insistence on proverbs and their unsuitability:

"Observe, Sancho," replied Don Quixote, "I bring in proverbs to the purpose, and when I quote them they fit like a ring to the finger; thou bringest them in by the head and shoulders, in such a way that thou dost drag them in, rather than introduce them; if I am not mistaken, I have told thee already that proverbs are short maxims drawn from the experience and observation of our wise men of old; but the proverb that is not to the purpose is a piece of nonsense and not a maxim."

(Part II, Chapter LXVII)

Don Quixote's observations reflect the difference in personalities between the two characters. Sancho is the archetype of a pragmatic and down to earth person, in direct opposition to his master, the eternally unsatisfied romantic dreamer. It is almost as if Don Quixote were asking his squire to go beyond those proverbs that end up being meaningless if not used appropriately. The novel's protagonist presents himself before Sancho as the great darer, someone who daydreams without measuring its consequences because imagination is beyond reality's determinations. Incidentally, the reader may find in the quote that Cervantes proposes a definition of "proverb"—reiterated several times throughout the book—which would be very suitable to refer to common place.

Perspective

To sum up, *deviants of thought* offer a false protection—a depersonalized protection—which from the beginning individuals have endeavored to put aside, knowing that they cannot guarantee not being inhabited themselves by those devices that lead all of life's colors to greys.

Readers may question the use of these considerations, which suggest a perspective that includes maturescence. Nevertheless, there is a reason that goes beyond a simple exegetical perspective. Maturescence is a great opportunity to let go of *common sense* in order to obtain one's *own individual sense*. Likewise, it is a chance to transform *common places* into *one's own individual place*, not only with regard to thought, but also from the perspective—experience?—of one's own life as from that moment; hopefully without euphemisms. Maturescence, then, would be a unique opportunity and an effort of personalization through this effort to obtain a direct comprehension of maturescence from an original indirect comprehension of maturescence.

Chapter 7

The mythical cycle of the hero (including Freud?)

In order to consider the human "invention" of aging, it is useful to compare the mythical cycle of the hero with the vital human cycle. Thus we find that adolescence and maturescence are perfectly typified and characterized as stages that the mythical hero undergoes in order to reach the personal growth that makes him fully human. This situation leads to a series of questions since it would confirm the proposals set forth by this author—following Freud (1910c) [p. 133] (1912c) [p. 235] (1916–1917 [1915–1917]) [p. 402] (1937c) [p. 226]—regarding how the pubertal and climacteric drive increases promote a kind of universal psychic work sufficiently important so as to be represented in the mythical productions of humanity.

It is therefore strangely paradoxical that the word "myth" is often used and understood to mean "lie" or "mistake." This may be just a paradox because anthropological, linguistic, and psychoanalytic studies of myths have demonstrated that they transmit profound, ancestral, and important truths, or what is most authentic about a particular culture. In the present case, myth accounts for the series of somatic processes that make evident the belonging of human beings to nature: puberty and climacterics as the moments in which the reproductive instinct is activated or reduced.

Of course, Freud already demonstrated that mythical truths are expressed through a process equivalent to dream work. Just as the manifest content of dreams uses apparently inconsequential day residues to disguise and express the actual latent content of dreams—always unattainable, incomprehensible and so heart-rending that it can bury itself in its own navel—myth work is based on an identical logic. But in this case, myths are "dreams of humankind." Such extreme efforts to mask and yet preserve their purpose with considerations of representativeness suggest that myths transmit truths that defy our ability to represent them.

Moreover, we could classify myths into two categories: the ones that attempt to explain the origin of the world and its ultimate fate, and the mythical cycle of the hero, usually concerned with the mysteries of life and death. Given that psychoanalysis acknowledges that universal psychic phenomena have mythical equivalents—for example, Oedipus and Narcissus—it is tempting to inquire how the characteristics peculiar to maturescence are expressed in the myth of the hero, adding another dimension to its definition.

Indeed, this proposal suggests that just as the exogamous departure that typifies adolescence is often contained in the heroic myth cycle dealing with the initiation ordeals that the hero must negotiate so as to be considered an adult member of society (departure); the particular vicissitudes (arrival) of maturescence appear in the period known as catabasis (return), or more specifically, "the Descent into Hell." It is at this moment that the hero undergoes a series of ordeals that make him "human."

A similar notion can be found in Nietzsche's *Also Sprach Zarathustra*—taking into account a tenet deriving from philosophy. The German concept termed *Untergung* denotes whims of fate, decadence, a descent aimed at personal insight coming from a reunion with the "origins" or with life's foundations.

During "the Descent into Hell," the hero often encounters his dead ancestors; he traverses some impenetrable, dark forest, makes a nocturnal journey, rescues a symbolic object that provides him with new insight, and so on. The upshot of all this can be his return home with new knowledge about life, with something valuable to be shared with others, with a kind of legacy, characterizing a process which we have named maturescence.

For these reasons, we have summarized certain aspects of the myths of Gilgamesh, Odysseus and Oedipus. Furthermore, we will consider some ideas regarding the life of Freud himself, our "hero" as psychoanalysts.

Gilgamesh

Specifically, in the anonymous Mesopotamian myth contained in the Gilgamesh saga—first epic poem and the most ancient literary work known so far—the hero begins "the descent into Hell" trying to find a formula or herb for "his" immortality. The "his" here emphasizes the strictly individual and narcissistic nature of this search because the impersonal allusion to the "herb of immortality" avoids admitting that the hero first seeks the formula for his own benefit, rather than for the benefit of the entire community, which will be the end result.

Written in cuneiform characters on clay tablets, the epic poem of Gilgamesh remained buried among the remains of the Asurbanipal Library for more than three thousand years. Moreover, repeated fires caused by the different invasions and conquests of the area, together with continuous floods, gave the mud a terracotta aspect. Damrosch (2006) states:

> Many tablets had been baked, giving them a heft and durability of terracotta roofing tiles, but most of them had been broken amid the ruins of Nineveh, so the collection consisted in a myriad of fragments.
>
> [p. 19]

Once the puzzle was put in place, the time for unveiling its meaning arrived. The interpretation of cuneiform writing took many years until it was possible to decipher it. The result was the discovery of the most beautiful poem ever known after having been preserved in the shadows: saved from floods, destruction and the encryption in a dead language, Gilgamesh surprised humanity after three thousand years of silence and unawareness of its existence.

The myth narrates the moving story of the king of Uruk, also known as Gilgamesh—two-thirds god and only one-third human—known for his cruelty and sadism. His conduct was so violent that the gods, tired and concerned about his unpredictability and the consequences of his acts on the people, decided to send an emissary with all the attributes necessary to defeat and kill him. Enkidu—two thirds human and only one third god—arrived at Uruk's kingdom and challenged Gilgamesh to a hand-to-hand combat, which finally ends in friendship between the two rivals. A warm, sincere and profound relationship ensues between them, a true archetype of friendship. One becomes the other's mirror, as they authentically understanding each other. So much so that together they decide to set off on a journey in search of extreme adventures for which they feel specially endowed. Without realizing it, their friendship had succeeded in defeating the design of the gods. At this point, Damrosch (2009) states, "Gilgamesh's thirst for adventure is fueled by a sense of the brevity and futility of life" [p. 209], as can be seen throughout the poem.

Informed and outraged by the failure of their objective by means of their emissary, the gods decide to do justice in a different way punishing Enkidu with death. This occurrence greatly upsets Gilgamesh who takes care of his dying friend until the last moments of his life, experiencing first hand from that moment the meaning of human suffering—let us remember that he is partly human by nature.

Unable to find solace, Gilgamesh decides to consult the only wise immortal that existed in the kingdom so that he could obtain eternal life, since he cannot tolerate the idea of death. In this case, Gilgamesh admits that he cannot tolerate the idea of "his" own death, since he has always considered himself immortal. Lamenting the death of his friend, he begs him to grant him immortality because he had never imagined the pain that death represents. Neither had he considered the pain of imagining himself dead. Unfortunately, the wise man tells him that he cannot grant him his wish since he himself ignores the reasons of his own immortality and that of his wife. Thus, he is unable to carry out his request: he supposes that it is something that occurred only once during the flood, but he is unable to help him. Nevertheless, the wife takes pity on Gilgamesh and suggests to the wise man that if he cannot grant him everlasting life, perhaps he could show him how to find the herb of eternal youth. Even if not quite the same, at least it will guarantee that he will not age, and Gilgamesh feels comforted. In order to obtain it, as it usually happens in most myths and also in ordinary life, the hero has to overcome a series of obstacles that make his objective difficult to attain. Gilgamesh finds the plant and commences his journey home. His transformation has been complete: he decides to bring the herb of immortality for all his people, not for himself, thus transforming "his" initial wish for eternal life into the wish for "our" immortality.

Before long and exhausted by the effort, Gilgamesh decides to rest for a moment. While he sleeps, a serpent eats the plant of immortality, instantly mutating into a youth that it had long lost. When Gilgamesh awakes, he understands what has happened: everything had been in vain. He then cries for what he realizes has been impossible: he would be one more among men, destined to die like any other human being. This realization, however, makes him even more human, mutating into a tolerant and sympathetic being, the just and fair king which he had never been up to then.

The epic poem raises the human dilemma of death starting from the conscious recognition during the maturescent process. Gilgamesh's process—a kind of "descent into Hell"—allows him to return home with a new knowledge of life, with something valuable to be shared with others, with a kind of legacy, as this author has previously suggested. For this reason, we can consider Gilgamesh as "the one who saw the abyss" [p. 4], as Gardner and Maier (1984) maintain in the introduction to the poem's translation, another suitable metaphor in order to understand the processing work of maturescence.

Gilgamesh's struggle with Enkidu could represent the encounter with his double—always a maturescent uncanny experience—which initiates the recognition process of his own individual death. It should be noted that this is something that occurs during Gilgamesh's adult life; that is, from the moment he commences his own "descent into Hell." In this peculiar aspect of the myth, we can infer the psychic processing that makes maturescence evident as well as the acquisition of wisdom of the concomitant life, in the same way that the quest for adventure characterizes the pubertal processing that leads to adolescence.

Odysseus

The concept of death sustained by the inhabitants of Ancient Greece can be inferred in many of their myths. Vernant (1996b) proposes that:

> As portrayed in epic, where it occupies a central position, Greek death appears disconcerting. It has two contrary faces. The first face is a glorious one: death shines out as the ideal to which the true hero devotes his existence. With its second face, death embodies the unsayable, the unbearable; it manifests itself as a terrifying horror.
>
> [p. 55]

In *The Odyssey*, the ancient Greek epic poem attributed to Homer, Odysseus (Ulysses), the King of Ithaca, was very reluctant to participate in the Trojan war— perhaps for representing these antithetical aspects of death alluded to by Vernant: happy in his kingdom, with his wife Penelope and his son Telemachus, he feigned madness when he was summoned to fight. Nevertheless, he was not able to deceive the authorities and had no choice but to participate in the conflict. Despite his initial reluctance, however, Odysseus became one of the war's most important heroes: honored and venerated as a warrior, he commenced his return journey with the glory of many accomplished feats that lead him to the urgency of a working-through for which he was not entirely prepared. Perhaps this explains why his return to Ithaca was delayed and hampered from the very beginning. In fact, it took Ulysses ten years to return home.

Up to what point can this delay be only associated to misfortunes or the role of *fate*—from the Latin *fatalis* "related to fateful, mortal," which in turn derives from *fatum* "destiny"—characteristic of a return, or does it express another conflict?

Odysseus wishes to return (manifest content) and laments the misfortunes (latent content) that cause his delay. In several instances, he cries with nostalgia for his kingdom and family; however, we can also surmise a certain ambivalence regarding his return.

Can we consider this conflict as an expression of the tensions that are characteristic of maturescence?

During the voyage home, Odysseus has intense relationships with several women that could be considered the archetypes of a certain kind of psychic functioning, representative of processes that can be activated during maturescence, as has been already described. Some of these female characters include Kalypso (a goddess–nymph), Athena (a true goddess), and his wife Penelope (a mortal).

Odysseus stays with Kalypso, a devastatingly beautiful goddess–nymph, for seven years. She is an egocentric, dominating nymph who holds him captive with the hope of marrying him. Vernant describes his predicament:

> But so long as he remains secluded and hidden with Kalipso, Odysseus' state is neither that of the living nor that of the dead. Although still alive, he is already (and ahead of time) like someone blotted out from human memory
>
> (Vernant, 1996b) [p. 187]

When he resists and is liberated by Hermes under orders from Zeus, Kalypso offers him immortality if he remains. Vernant (1996b), again:

> If he agrees to remain with her, she promises to make him immortal and to spare him forever from old age and death. He will live in her company as a god, immortal, in the permanent bloom of youth, for never to die and never to know the decrepitude of old age are what one stands to gain from love shared with the goddess.
>
> [p. 188]

But Odysseus, after many doubts, painfully declines the offer:

> The Kalipso episode presents, for the first time in our literary tradition, what might be called the heroic refusal of immortality.
>
> [p. 188]

Odysseus' decision can be considered heroically authentic, since he decides to renounce immortality to promote a certain heroic immortality that can lead to the fulfillment of his desire: Penelope and Telemachus. This renunciation of immortality can be considered equivalent to what was previously suggested when we discussed the epic of Gilgamesh.

Psychoanalytically speaking, Kalypso may be regarded as an object that facilitated the expression of the ideal ego: predominance of the pleasure principle dissociated from the reality principle, and Odysseus triumphs over the ideal ego trying to be near his ego ideal. His refusal "leads him at last to find death desirable" (Vernant, 1996b) [p. 189].

However, Odysseus also loves Penelope, Telemachus and his kingdom. Some critics dismiss Penelope as a paragon of marital fidelity—a serious and industrious character, a devoted wife and mother. But Penelope is in a very dangerous situation when the suitors begin invading her house, asking—and then demanding—her hand in marriage. Her son, Telemachus, has neither the maturity nor the strength to expel the invaders. Although unassuming, Penelope has a cunning that indicates she is a good mate for her wily husband.

The story of the loom symbolizes the queen's clever tactics. For three years, Penelope worked at weaving a shroud for the eventual funeral of her father-in-law, Laertes. She claimed that she would choose a husband as soon as the shroud was completed. By day, the queen, a renowned weaver, worked on a great loom in the royal halls. At night, she secretly unraveled what she had done, amazingly deceiving the young suitors. Her ploy failed only when one of her servants eventually betrayed her and told the suitors what was happening.

After Odysseus returns to Ithaca, the queen announces to the visiting beggar, whom she suspects to be Odysseus, that she will hold a contest in which the suitors will be asked to string the great bow of Odysseus and shoot an arrow through a dozen axes, an old trick of her husband's, and that she will be the wife of the man who can perform the feat. The choice of this particular contest is no coincidence, since Penelope knows exactly what she is doing. If the old beggar really is Odysseus in disguise, he alone has any realistic chance of winning the contest.

The goddess Athena, for her part, is a consistent supporter of Odysseus, intervening repeatedly on behalf of the hero and his son, Telemachus. She often appears in disguise, most significantly as Mentor, the family friend and adviser who instructs Telemachus in his father's absence. She is also adept at changing the appearance of humans. When Odysseus returns to Ithaca and needs a disguise in order to gather information without revealing his true identity, Athena turns him into an old beggar, even wrinkling his skin and taking the fire out of his eyes. When appropriate, she renews his vigor, making him look taller, stronger and younger.

Athena's intervention is always essential, but she lets mortals earn their destinies. In the battle with the suitors, for example, she bestows just enough courage to Odysseus so as to help him turn the tide; but then she recedes into the background and allows mortals their victory.

This author would like to suggest that between these three women a tension is produced that evinces what Odysseus experiences. Kalypso promises immortality (ideal ego) [dissociation of the pleasure principle from the reality principle]; Athena functions like a positive internal object who manipulates the winds in favor of the hero so that he can fulfill his destiny [evidence of the psychic working-through]; and Penelope makes it possible to recuperate authentic satisfaction [fusion of the pleasure principle with the reality principle]. Odysseus solves the tension proposed by the three figures.

Nevertheless, if the plot of the return to Ithaca can be understood as a "descent into Hell," Odysseus also undergoes a specific "Descent into Hades"—equivalent to the "the descent into Hell"—on his way back to Ithaca from the Trojan War. He follows Circe's instructions to consult Tiresias about his future, deciding to follow his advice and return to his homeland. He traverses the straits of Scylla and Charybdis, cleverly survives the mermaids' songs and other dangerous obstacles until he finally returns home to his wife Penelope and his son Telemachus—just as Tiresias has predicted. Finley (1967) states:

> Odysseus will indeed reach home, says the seer. Returning home, he will rule in peace over a happy people and reach a shining old age, and a gentle death will come to him from the sea.
>
> [p. 355]

The power of The Odyssey resides in its allusion to this profoundly human theme, which permeates not only the original psychic structuring but also different moments of the life cycle, for example: the tensions of maturescence and the concomitant resolution.

Oedipus

Aristotle considered *Oedipus Rex* as the perfect tragedy. It contains the three elements that he considered essential for a tragic scheme: error (*hamartia*), recognition (*anagnórisis*) and change of fortune (*peripeteia*). García Gual (2012) maintains that:

> "The tragic adventure consists in the hero's change of fortune. At the beginning, he is at the height of his power. However, a sudden change occurs due

to his errors and his previous glory has a catastrophic outcome. Despite his achievements and nobleness, the protagonist seems doomed to a cruel death, or, as in the case of Oedipus, to a fierce punishment: blindness and exile."

[p. 122]

We could perhaps consider that Oedipus's punishment is the result of wanting to know and understand the truth. This recognition is what this author considers Oedipus's "descent into Hell": the effort to solve his enigmatic origins in order to reach a level of development that is above the human median. García Gual (2012) further points out:

The fatality of destiny is no longer presented as a basic lesson, the fulfillment of the oracle. Instead, it serves as a warning of how the search for truth and the desire for knowledge leads the noble Oedipus to catastrophe. Because of his magnanimous character, he will not be influenced by the advice of those who try to turn him away from his dangerous enquiries, which finally lead to a disastrous outcome. Man's "radical insecurity" is what drags heroes to their doom.

[p. 129]

But Oedipus is also a "deregulated" myth, as Goux (1999) maintains—a myth that follows a path different from the rest, since the initiatory order is inverted. In fact, Oedipus is "initiated" when he decides to leave Corinth. The first time he consulted the oracle, he was told that he would assassinate his father. In order to avoid that destiny, he left the city where he supposed his father lived. This event could have taken place around Oedipus's puberty.

Long after he killed his father, when he manages to work out the enigma of the Sphinx—a sufficiently amazing feat that results in the Sphinx's immediate suicide—he is proclaimed king of Thebes and marries Jocasta, the wife of king Laius, who is in fact Oedipus's real mother, unbeknown to both mother and son. For this reason, this author maintains that the authentic initiation, with all its sexual connotations, occurs when Oedipus solves the Sphinx's enigma. He then takes up residence and has children with his own mother. He reigns in peace and harmony, respected by his subjects, until the plague breaks out in Thebes. Then the city is subjected to famine, infirmity and death. Ignoring the reasons why Thebes is ravaged by such a powerful tragedy, Oedipus consults Tiresias—once more the official soothsayer—who always facilitated Oedipus's search to discover his origins, his authentic "descent into Hell." García Gual (1981) sustains:

Oedipus and Tiresias represent two powers, the King vis-à-vis the soothsayer, and the confrontation, with all its tragic irony, unveils the superiority of the blind soothsayer over the highly intelligent monarch ... The blind fortune teller moves in the frontier of two worlds. With his eyes closed to the world where he puts his feet, a clumsy walker, he can glimpse into the future. This opposition between the visible and the invisible translates to the one between life and death.

[p. 170]

The emblematic tragedy by Sophocles contains some aspects of the indispensable psychic working-through entailed by maturescence. The play describes some of Oedipus's earlier consultations with the oracle, whose pronouncements the hero has disdained. As a result, this author wonders why Oedipus was unable to discover his origins earlier. Why did events have to culminate in "the plague" in order to consult the oracle that led him to the knowledge he was searching for? Oedipus's self-discovery is his own "Descent into Hell," the sort of "plague" (return of the repressed?) that is typical of maturescence.

Macbeth's marriage and the curse of sterility

Although *Macbeth* is a tragedy instead if a myth, one might think that, since the loss of fertility is so important throughout the process here depicted, people who have had children would be better off than those who did not. However, psychoanalytic clinical data seem to refute this. Regardless of whether people have had children or not, they will go through this unconscious subject because it is something that becomes a worry that will activate itself somatically, just as the referred myths show.

Here once again, psychopathology provides the opportunity to magnify those processes which, in balanced states, could go unnoticed. Regarding these data and aware that only one issue within a complex and multi-vocal work of art is being raised, this author will now address parts of *Macbeth*'s plot by William Shakespeare.

As Freud himself points out (1916d), Macbeth's marriage would end up in an extreme diffusion of drives owing to infertility. In this context it is often surprising to read Freud's declaration that Macbeth's marriage is "a demonstration of the curse of unfruitfulness and the blessings of continuous generation" (p. 320). The words "curse" and "blessings" come as a surprise, since Freud was not prone to use metaphors in this way.

Having failed in nature's "plan," King Macbeth understands that he will have no descendants and his throne will be headless. That was the message predestined by the Three Witches, resembling the three Fates of classical mythology. So one might think that since the couple fails to fulfill the "plan" of nature (or will no longer be able to fulfill it), they embark on the serial, murderous, and bloody stratagem in order to process drive increase confronted with the background of the underlying aphanisis that characterizes maturescence; the situation condemns them to become simple "mortals."

From the perspective this author proposes, it is possible to imagine that the King and Queen commit murder not because they fail to pass on the germ-plasm without the "blessings of continuous generations," but because they have no psychic resources to work-through this specific post-climacteric process. Even if they had had children, the couple perhaps would have suffered the same despair and violence, which might have been displaced to some other situations sufficiently unimportant so as to hide their true pain of no longer being biologically necessary. With greater psychic resources, there is a greater likelihood of working-through this moratorium than in the absence of genetic or symbolic offspring, but the lack of these resources would bring about a diffusion of drives similar to what the Macbeths experienced.

Freud?

Likewise, with the interpretation of *Oedipus Rex* described above, one cannot help but conclude that Freud's own destiny was similar to that of Oedipus, since he discovered the Oedipus complex when he commenced his self-analysis: when he began his personal and own "Descent into Hell."

It would seem that in the heroic myths, Gilgamesh, Odysseus, Oedipus, and in the one related to our "hero" Freud, one finds a "Descent into Hell" that evinces the psychic work of maturescence which, according to Freud (1915b), "compels us once more to be heroes who cannot believe in their own death" [p. 299]. This specific psychic work simultaneously obliges us to make the conscious effort to acknowledge inevitable personal death. Of course, this conceptualization also entails the tenet which maintains that—following Freud, 1921c)—"the hero was a man who by himself had slain the father: the father who still appeared in the myth as a totemic monster" [p. 136]. This act is actually the subjective authorization for adulthood and adulthood's consequent maturescence.

Freud himself maintained that he commenced his self-analysis as a consequence of the death of his father in October, 1896. Anzieu (1986), putting into practice Jaques's model, proposes a profound and surprising reading of Freud's midlife crisis, postulating the commencement of Freud's self-analysis previous to the death of his father. He maintains:

> Ever since the spring of 1894, when, as we have seen, Freud experienced heart trouble that was made more acute by nicotine poisoning, he had been familiar with the fear of dying and aware of the inevitability of his own death.
>
> [p. 165]

> At the same time Freud was beginning to think about death, as is inevitable at an age when we realise we have entered the second half of our lives.
>
> [p. 117]

> In the middle of 1895, Freud began to enter his mid-life crisis. That crisis was superactivated, from the autumn of 1896 on, by the work of mourning.
>
> [p. 211]

The three examples quoted above coincide with Jaques's model (1965) to understand the midlife crisis—different from the one suggested by this author.

Soon after the death of his father, Freud wrote to Fliess, in September, 1896:

> I write to you today because an influenza with fever, suppuration and heart discomfort suddenly broke my well-being; but starting from today I detect some kind of recovery. I would gladly prefer to reach the famous age limit circa 51, although there was a day when I thought this highly improbable.
>
> [p. 210]

Here another episode commences because Freud—we might add, fortunately—does not escape the common neurosis that afflicts all human beings. We could therefore consider that Anzieu's interpretation of Freud's midlife crisis would simply imply his entry to full adult life—what this author calls indirect understanding of maturescence. Somehow the concept of midlife crisis proposed by Jaques, seen retroactively after so many years, can be considered as an evolutionary stage that proposes access to adult fulfillment—a stage of the vital cycle prior to maturescence—considering that the authentic midlife crisis would imply the kind of maturescent process suggested by this author. Freud continues worrying about death, which leads to the discovery of another transcendental nodal point as he reaches his fiftieth birthday, an aspect that could be significant to future biographers of his life and work, from the point of view of maturescence.

Consistent with Fliess's periodicity theory, which attributed repetitive circuits of 23 (for men) and 28 (for women)—cycles that in turn predestined the date of birth, illness and death—Freud begins to worry about his own fifty-first birthday: $23 + 28 = 51$, considering this as the future date of his own death. Anzieu (1986) asserts that:

> Fliess had worked out that his friend would reach a critical point in his life at the age of 51 (28 + 23, i.e. a male cycle + a female cycle). It was the age Freud feared he would die.
>
> [p. 438]

Fifteen years before he reached that age, while interpreting an absurd dream of a dead father, Freud (1900a), writing *The Interpretation of Dreams*, had already stated:

> However, the number 51 by itself, without the number of the century, was determined in another, and indeed, in an opposite sense; and this, too, is why it appeared in the dream several times. 51 is the age which seems to be a particularly dangerous one to men; I have known colleagues who have died suddenly at that age, and amongst them one who, after long

delays, had been appointed to a professorship only a few days before his death.

[p. 438]

This was reinforced by a certain Jewish mystical belief that places a fateful tone on the number 52, leading us to consider that it is a critical age for men. Schur (1972) affirms:

The number 52 could be spelled out as the Hebrew word for dog—hence a bad number—and the 52nd birthday was considered a "critical" one, especially for men.

[p. 25]

Jones (1955) describes a curious scene that took place during Freud's fiftieth birthday:

In 1906, on the occasion of his fiftieth birthday, the little group of adherents in Vienna presented him with a medallion, having on the obverse his side-portrait in bas-relief and on the reverse a Greek design of Oedipus answering the Sphinx. Around it is a line from Sophocles' *Oedipus Tyrannus*: "Who divined the famed riddle and was a man most mighty." At the presentation of the medallion there was a curious incident. When Freud read the inscription he became pale and agitated and in a strangled voice demanded to know who had thought of it. He behaved as if he had encountered a *revenant*, and so he had. After Federn told him it was he who had chosen the inscription, Freud disclosed that as a young student at the University of Vienna he used to stroll around the great Court inspecting the busts of former famous professors of the institution. He then had the fantasy, not merely of seeing his own bust there in the future, which would not have been anything remarkable in an ambitious student, but of it actually being inscribed with the *identical words* he now saw on the medallion.

[vol II, p. 15]

Schur continues (1972):

Freud disliked such celebrations where arbitrarily chosen dates—decade, or later half-decade marks—were made occasions for special attention. Nonetheless he viewed as a special feat one's having wrested another few years away from death or from "inexorable Ananke", as he would later call it, while at the same time having overcome the "burden of existence" and the "exigencies of life."

[p. 244]

And although after 1904 he repeatedly expressed his resentment about aging, he did so with some exaggeration but apparently without any obsessive preoccupation with dying after the acute upsurge of that year. This held true even in 1907 when Freud reached the "fateful" and "critical" age of 28 + 23.

[p. 244]

For these reasons, perhaps we could conceive of the existence of a maturescent process around this period in Freud's life—which would radically change Anzieu's perspective—that extends its scope until it reaches Freud's fiftieth year as a nodal point in order to find a style of processing typical of maturescence that could also perhaps be found in his theoretical production.

Chapter 8

Background

It was already mentioned that there is a great deal of psychoanalytical literature about middle age—often sustaining that the so-called mid-life crisis is the origin of a period of the lifecycle also known as midlife (middle age?), something no so clear.

The concept *maturescence* is a neologism proposed and coined by this author, through the translation of his paper on *madurescencia*—the corresponding word in Spanish—which was published by *The International Journal of Psycho-Analysis* (2015). The term does not appear in previous studies; it is suggested as a specificity that permits a meta-psychological understanding based on a strictly Freudian conceptualization.

Stages for the definition of the midlife concept

The midlife concept and its related studies have a history that could be divided into various stages:

- The August Weismann legacy.
- First definition of midlife (1965).
- Psychological definition of midlife (1930–1965).
- First studies (1970–2000).
- Psychoanalytic works by Calvin Anthony Colarusso.
- Absence of research and contributions by this author (Montero) (2001–2010).
- Other studies.
- Miscellany.
- Five questions for a survey about midlife (2009).
- Research carried out by this author (Montero) (2011–2018).
- Current non–psychoanalytic investigations.

The August Weismann legacy

The unexpected precursor whose perspective intended to propose a state of the art on this subject is August Weismann (1834–1914). Freud supported several of his theoretical concepts. Weismann was a German biologist who held that acquired characteristics are not transmitted to one's progeny. This theory was in direct opposition to *the inheritance of acquired characteristics* sustained by Lamarck (1744–1829).

Weismann, who did not delve into psychological topics, could be considered the pioneer of a whole line of thinkers that have contributed to the theme of the somatic impact on psychic life. In fact, he considered germ-plasm as an essentially *immortal* substance, since it is transmitted from one organism to another through reproduction. In addition, he suggested that a soma, which brings the rest of an organism together, would be a mere vehicle for the transmission of germ-plasm. This process, known as the Weismann barrier, sustains that hereditary information is only transmitted from germline cells to somatic cells, never the other way around.

Freud (1920g) takes up Weismann's ideas:

> It was (Weismann) who introduced the division of living substance into mortal and immortal parts. The mortal part is the body in the narrower sense—the "soma"—which alone is subject to natural death. The germ-cells, on the other hand, are potentially immortal, in so far as they are able, under certain favorable conditions, to develop into a new individual, or, in other words, to surround themselves with a new soma ... Weismann, regarding living substance morphologically, sees in it one portion which is destined to die—the soma, the body apart from the substance concerned with sex and inheritance—and an immortal portion—the germ-plasm, which is concerned with the survival of the species, with reproduction.
>
> [p. 46]

These propositions also led Freud (1914c) [p. 78] (1915c) [p. 125] (1916–1917 [1915–1917]) [p. 316] (1920g) [p. 45] (1933a [1932]) [p. 95] to his concept of the double existence of human beings, already mentioned in the chapter *Psychoanalysis of maturescence: the onset of middle age and beyond.* For example, Freud (1914c) sustains:

> The individual does actually carry on a twofold existence: one to serve his own purposes and the other as a link in a chain, which he serves against his will, or at least involuntarily. The individual himself regards sexuality as one of his own ends; whereas from another point of view he is an appendage to his germ-plasm, at whose disposal he puts his energies in return of a bonus of pleasure. He is the mortal vehicle of a (possible) immortal substance—like the inheritor of an entailed property, who is only the temporary holder of an estate which survives him.
>
> [p. 78]

Many years later, Richard Dawkins (1976) returns to the same idea when he suggests that human conduct is rooted in biological bases, similarly to Weisman's theory. He suggests the concept of *replicator* as an equivalent of gene and the *survival machine* as an equivalent of soma. His proposal overturns the theory of evolution, since the focus of his theory would cease to be the preservation of the species but rather the preservation of the gene as the ultimate and indivisible unit. A line of continuity is thus suggested, from Weismann and including Freud, which culminates with Dawkins and his followers.

This theoretical perspective allows us to infer the great importance of somatic processes in psychic development. For example, it could be considered that the ideas of immortality, so common in the human species—the search and desire of immortality could represent metaphorically the reality of this form of continuity of life—could be sustained in this double constitution of human nature alluded by Freud, and could be considered the expression of a subjective perception of this *immortality* of substance, whether we call it germ-plasm, gene or whatever term adopted in future for this biological characteristic and its impact on psychic life.

First definition of midlife in psychoanalysis (1965)

The first time that a partially equivalent concept of middle age appears in psychoanalytical literature, it does so as mid-life crisis. In his work *Death and the Mid-Life Crisis* (1965), Elliott Jaques puts forward the concept of mid-life crisis. For the record, we would like to make it clear that the concept of midlife as this book tries to explain it does not appear in the above-mentioned work. Even though the abstract of Jaques's article seems directly related to this topic, surprisingly the author does not refer to it later on. In fact, his final assertions there seem to differ from his own thesis because in the abstract starting the paper he sustains that:

> The transition is often obscured in women by the proximity of the onset of changes connected with the menopause. In the case of men, the change has from time to time been referred to as male climacteric, because of the reduction in the intensity of sexual behaviour which often occurs at that time.
>
> (Jaques, 1965) [p. 502]

But the fact that Jaques, throughout this work, does not refer to female and male climacteric is really surprising. It could be surmised that what was published as the abstract in *The International Journal of Psychoanalysis* was not written by him but by those who edited the paper. If this would have been Jaques's purpose, then his work would undoubtedly be a forerunner of the concept of *maturescence* this book puts forward. But it didn't happen this way.

Analyzing the paper's content, Jaques suggests a crisis that occurs during midlife, sustaining that it commences at about thirty-five years of age. However, both menopause and andropause occur much later in human biological evolution. Secondly, both phenomena are not necessarily related to a supposed reduction of either sexual conduct or sexual desire. In fact, it could be maintained, from a meta-psychological perspective, that exactly the opposite takes place. Both menopause and andropause increase psychic work. The latter seems to be linked to a drive increase stemming from menopause and andropause, confronted by each individual according to his internal organization.

Jaques carries out a Kleinian study of what he suggests as mid-life crisis, using as a starting point an analysis of the change he observes in artistic creativity. He argues that when creative individuals become approximately thirty-five years old, a change occurs in the manner, quality and content of creative work that distinguishes early adulthood from mature adulthood, as he terms these two different stages of life. On the basis of his studies of the creativity of several artists, he sustains that during early adulthood, creativity is characterized by exaltation, spontaneity and urgency. In contrast, during mature adulthood, a sculptural creativity takes place, characterized by a much more reflexive and elaborative style and content.

Furthermore, Jacques maintains that, during the mid-life crisis, a reprocessing of the depressive position is worked again in the Kleinian sense. This would motivate, in turn, the change in the type of creativity and the onset of an individual's acknowledgement of his own future death. In this way, he suggests that a working-through of the Kleinian paranoid–schizoid position would appear during adolescence. In the mid-life crisis, on the other hand, something similar would take place with the depressive position—precisely that which could onset the frequent depressive crises, activated during this stage of life:

> With the awareness of the onset of the last half of life, unconscious depressive anxieties are aroused, and the repetition and continuation of the working-through of infantile depressive position are required.
>
> (Jaques, 1965) [p. 511]

Thus, Jaques would be proposing a link between adolescence and mid-life, although not to the point of conceptualizing the (peri)climacteric drive increase that characterizes maturescence.

This thesis could coincide with the affirmation that the mid-life crisis is activated when the individual has completed his biological development and begins to age:

> The paradox is that of entering the prime of life, the stage of fulfilment, but at the same time the prime and fulfilment are dated. Death lies beyond.
>
> (Jaques, 1965) [p. 506]

Relying on Freud (1915b), Jaques considers that this occurs when an individual begins to comprehend that death has now become a personal matter:

> The compulsive attempts, in many men and women reaching middle age, to remain young, the hypochondriacal concern over health and appearance, the emergence of sexual promiscuity in order to prove youth and potency, the hollowness and lack of genuine enjoyment of life, and the frequency of religious concern, are familiar patterns. They are attempts at a race against time.
>
> (Jaques, 1965) [p. 511]

According to Jaques, this reactive symptom would make evident a certain emotional impoverishment that impedes confronting the anxieties of early adulthood that would enable the individual to enjoy life in a truly mature way. In addition, he proposes the concept of *constructive resignation* as a synthesis of the type of proactive psychic work that this stage of early adulthood demands.

Even though Jaques's work became a mandatory reference for subsequent works, providing a very good Kleinian meta-psychological description of what he calls *mid-life crisis*—a concept that has earned its place—it is surprising that he places it in what could be termed early adulthood.

Jaques's ideas seem to lack the intermediate concept of mid-adulthood because it establishes an early adulthood and a late adulthood, as if he were describing processes that are much more related to early adulthood than mid-adulthood. Finally, Jaques's work also found continuity in the works of Segal (1984) and Waddell (1998).

Psychological definition of midlife (1930–1965)

The real forerunner of psychological studies—not psychoanalytic—about midlife was Carl Gustav Jung (1930). In his work *The decline of life* he sustains what could be considered a first approach to the midlife theme. He considers that an individual who gets old has the obligation to take care of his internal world—which would exclude young people. The internal process Jung postulates, starting from what he terms the midday of life, is the process of individuation: the conquest of one's internal world, which would start at approximately forty years of age. In addition, he suggests an introversion of the libido, typical of this stage of life, as opposed to the extraversion of the first half of life. This would explain why the second half of one's life could not be guided by the same principles as the first, according to the cited reference.

In a similar manner, Jolande Jacobi (1939)—exegete of Jung—proposes two moments of individuation that entail an enantiodromia; that is, a change of sign *between* these two stages, something that could happen in midlife.

Analytic psychology, as Jung's psychology is known by, also has a specific study about midlife by Murray Stein (1983), *In Midlife: A Jungian Perspective*. This author proposes that midlife is a moment in which individuals experience a fundamental change in their alignment with life and the world. This change has a psychological and religious significance, regardless of its interpersonal and social dimensions. Therefore, the author considers midlife as a spiritual crisis.

After Jung, and many years before Jaques, the first draft of a definition concerning midlife as the starting point of middle age within the psychoanalytic field, can be found in Erik Erikson (1951). In order to explain the developmental stages of the ego, he suggests eight stages of human life. The seventh stage, *generativity versus stagnation*, would correspond to the psychic work of midlife, even though he does not refer to the alluded period in this way.

Erikson sustains that the fear of death is the consequence of a lack of ego integration, which he defines as an accumulated security, a kind of post-narcissistic love, or a love that goes beyond narcissism; the acceptance of a unique cycle of life that each individual must experience. Only after this ego consolidation does death change its significance, losing its tormenting aspect. In this way, he proposes *wisdom* as the true and basic virtue of this stage of life; that which can be perceived as a consequence of this ego integration.

A great psychoanalyst, not as well-known as Jaques despite having been one of Freud's assistants in Vienna during the 1930s, was Edmund Bergler. In his book, *The Revolt of the Middle Aged Man* (1954), he proposes a definition that deserves to be considered. He argues that midlife is a *revolt against biology*. This phrase could include the psychological aspect: midlife is a (psychological) revolt against biology's mandate; a powerful metaphor that synthesizes a large part of this book's intention. Unfortunately, he does not go deeper into the somatic implications of the phrase, which could have functioned as a preview of a comprehension equivalent to the one postulated with maturescence. Nevertheless, he sustains that this *revolt* could be considered as a second adolescence, together with a marked hypochondria. Perhaps this author could object to Bergler's view for suggesting a kind of psychopathology of midlife; a *revolt* would imply a pathological state in itself. Nevertheless, he is the true pioneer and exegete of the concept of midlife, even if Jaques and his successors did not take him into account.

First studies (1970–2000)

Erikson's works preceded the pscychoanalytical studies of Spitz, Anna Freud and Mahler, who laid the foundations of the studies related to the life cycle beyond adolescence; they maintained an epigenetic and evolutionist perspective of psychic development, paving the way for a specific understanding of mid-life. These authors proposed the continuity of psychic development beyond childhood and adolescence, including the different stages of libidinal evolution: oral, phallic and genital. Their research enabled studies related to adult life, middle age and old age—a true revolution that opened doors to a re-signification of the human life cycle.

René A. Spitz (1965) distinguishes maturity from development. He proposes that maturity is the display of the species' functions. This is the result of the phylogenetic evolution that emerges in the course of embryonic development or is transmitted after birth, like *anlage*, in later stages of life. On the other hand, development implies the apparition of forms, functions and conducts that are the result of the interchange between the organism and its internal and external environment.

What is important for the current study of maturescence is that Spitz also focuses on development, when he describes the series of organizers which are affective expressions indicating that a new level of psychic organization and structuring has been reached. He considers that development is cumulative as well as epigenetic; in other words, each development level is built upon a previous one. Then, this author could suggest an organizer for each critical stage of development, sometimes he has therefore postulated, together with Colarusso (Montero & Colarusso) (2007), a specific organizer for midlife called *adult psychic organizer*.

Spitz's conceptualization is very important because it evinces how biological maturity allows psychic development to *lean* on it, in the same sense that Freud suggested that sexual drives lean on self-preservation drives, in line with the concept of maturescence suggested in this study.

From the perspective of Ego-psychology, Anna Freud (1963) (1965) develops her concept of developmental lines whereby she represents the sequential progress, emphasizing the continuous and the cumulative character of development. She suggests a prototype of developmental lines that go from dependence to emotional self-sufficiency and the adult object relations as well as developmental lines towards corporal independence, among others. She also outlines a metapsychological profile of the adult that evaluates the different developmental lines, including drive and representational activity. This adult metapsychological profile provides a relevant precedent when we consider the psychic specificity of the adult up to mid-life.

From the perspective of the object relations theory, Margaret Mahler (1968) (1977) proposes the separation–individuation theory. Separation implies the process whereby the child gradually forms an intrapsychic representation of self, different and separated from the object representation. Individuation, on the other hand, refers to the child's attempts to develop a personal identity. She distinguishes between a normal autistic phase and a symbiotic autistic phase before the process of separation–individuation specifically commences. This process includes the following stages: differentiation, practicing, rapprochement and object constancy. It is worth considering that Mahler suggests that individuation is a process which encompasses the whole human life cycle; for this reason, she is included here.

In relation to the above but referring now to a psychological specificity of adult life, midlife and old age, the compiling effort of Greenspan and Pollock (1980) is an attempt to make a revision in a series of six volumes that offer theoretic and clinical evidence regarding the continuity and psychic development throughout the life cycle.

A few years later, Otto Kernberg (1980) details relevant features of narcissism, starting from Klein (1963) and Jaques (1965), when considering the *vital tasks* in midlife. In the chapter *Normal Narcissism in Middle Age*, he suggests the following features: a change in time perspective, an inversion in the rate of external and internal changes, the recognition of the limits of creativity, a modification of Ego identity in the perspective of time, the acknowledgement of external aggression, the presence of loss, bereavement and death and an updating of oedipal conflicts.

In the chapter *Pathological Narcissism in Middle Age*, he describes some of the typical defensive mechanisms of pathological narcissism. He maintains that a narcissistic patient is *eternally young*, not only in the sense of not being prepared to admit the passage of time, but because he internally lacks the possibility of accumulating an internal life that can provide the support and compensation for future losses and eventual failure. He links this issue with the difficulty of admitting old age. Kernberg does not suggest a specific metapsychology for midlife but rather seems to overlap what characterizes the narcissist patient with what occurs during middle age. Nevertheless, his work is an attempt to delve into the understanding of this period of life.

We would also like to consider the work of Hanna Segal (1984), framed within Jaques's line of thought. Segal applies the Kleinian model of psychoanalysis to two works by Joseph Conrad, *Heart of Darkness* (1899) and *The Shadow Line* (1916), attributing mid-life crisis issues to the novels' main characters. She maintains that Conrad's *shadow line* is a metaphor for that threshold that must be transposed in order to acquire an adult perspective of one's own subjectivity; and that the *heart of darkness*—through Kurtz, its main character—alludes to the profoundly incomprehensible essence of human nature and the impossibility of avoiding hate and aggression as founding roots of human nature.

Pearl King (1980) focuses on the transferential phenomena in treatments of middle age patients or those who have reached late adulthood. Freud (1912c), on the other hand, had begun his work considering how evolutionary biological processes (puberty and menopause) produced an alteration of the equilibrium of psychic processes—thematic nucleus of this theorization. However, Pearl King soon ignored this affirmation to pose the series of pressures to which patients within this age range are subjected, pressures which are the result of the impact generated by certain social and psychological aspects characteristic of adult life. Thus, she distanced herself towards destinies unrelated to his point of departure.

Pearl King proposes the fear of loss of sexual potency, the worry of being displaced from the workforce by younger candidates, the *empty nest* anxiety, the conscience of aging and the acknowledgement of the inevitability of individual's own death and the unfulfillment of desired projects, something which could lead to depressive states. This kind of reasoning is what is suggested in this book as an indirect understanding of maturescence, confusing what is overt from the authentic latent content.

Daniel Levinson also deserves special mention because he carried out an empirical study of the human life cycle from the perspective of a non-psychoanalytical, developmental psychology. He researched the life course of several men (1978) and women (1996) for many years, formalizing a stage which he named midlife.

For Levinson, the definition of life cycle includes two aspects. The first one encompasses the idea of process or voyage, from a starting point (birth, origin) up to a culmination point (death, conclusion). He attempts to demonstrate that the voyage from birth up to old age follows a universal subjacent pattern or a basic sequence that covers countless cultural and individual variations. The second aspect is the idea of *seasons of life* or series of stages within the life cycle, each one qualitatively different from its own distinctive character. He considers each season as a relatively stable segment of the life cycle, even though interconnected with each other during each transition period. Thus he poses the universality of a transition from midlife, between forty and forty-five years of age, period in which an individual would pass from early adulthood to mid-life.

Even though he is not a psychoanalyst, Levinson bases his theory on Winnicott (1971) to define his idea of transition. Adopting the latter's concept of illusion, he suggests that during the mid-life transition, a process takes place that would not imply a *disillusionment* but, instead, a *de-illusionment* (1978), a concept closer to what Jaques had proposed as *constructive resignation*, already alluded to.

Suggesting a system of stages and sub-stages that are articulated with each other, Levinson maintains that the *developmental task* of the mid-life transition implies modifying the life structure of early adulthood until it is transformed into a life structure that is appropriate to mid-life. He therefore poses four changes in the life structure during the mid-life transition (1996):

1. Change in sleeping habits (individual accomplishment).
2. Interaction with a mentor.
3. End of the occupation/profession setting.
4. Reformulation of love relationships

Finally, from the perspective of psychoanalysis, Franco de Masi (2002) alludes to life's transience, sustaining that the great problem of humanity is the awareness of its own mortality. Taking up Aeschylus' tragedy, de Massi suggests that Prometheus benefited humanity not by stealing fire from the gods but by denying humanity the knowledge of its own mortality. De Masi considers that Prometheus' gift was to give human beings the comforting liberty of living without pre-established time boundaries. De Masi's work is one of the few serious attempts that provide us with access to an understanding of the place mortality occupies in human psychic life.

The psychoanalytic works of Calvin Anthony Colarusso

Calvin Anthony Colarusso's work is made up of six thick volumes—five in English (three in collaboration with Robert A. Nemiroff as authors and editors and two of which he is the author) and one in Spanish; the latter compiling the translation of works published in different international magazines. All his works are related to exploring the different phases of the life cycle, especially centered on adult life, middle age and late adulthood.

Colarusso may be considered a developmental scholar, from the perspective of Anna Freud. For this reason, he takes up the concept of Anna Freud's developmental lines (1963) (1965), crossing them with Levinson's developmental tasks (1978) (1996). Colarusso suggests extending the developmental lines to old age, among which he describes the developmental line of the body and the developmental line of time and death (1999) (2000).

The series of midlife *tasks* he formulates—in consonance with Levinson (1978)—includes the acknowledgement of the *aging of the body* and the growing conscience of *time limitation* and *individual's own death*. Furthermore, when he proposes the seven hypotheses for a psychodynamic theory of adult development (1981), he maintains that one of these implies that adult development is profoundly influenced by the body and physical change, also suggesting that a central theme, specific in adult development, is the normative crisis brought about by the acknowledgement and acceptance of time limitation and the inevitability of personal death.

Colarusso places great importance in the loss phenomenon (loss of physical abilities, loss of neurons, loss of intelligence) to then highlight everything that humans still continue to acquire when changes in the body commence (neural growth, the role of glial cells, chemical modifications), but he does not seem to focus on the transformation of somatic stimuli in psychic phenomena.

In the book Colarusso compiles in 1985 regarding the second half of life, there is almost no mention of the psychic expression of the somatic issue. The same can be said of his 1990 work, where the authors invite other psychoanalysts to dedicate a chapter on the different decades of adulthood; the soma and the body, however, are practically not mentioned throughout the twenty chapters.

On the other hand, in *Child and Adult Development* (1992), Colarusso is much more explicit. The chapter he dedicates to midlife is eloquent because he once again suggests that the key developmental task of midlife implies the acceptance of the aging process of the body and the acknowledgment of time limitation and personal death, which he also upholds in *Fulfillment in Adulthood: Paths to the Pinnacle of Life* (1994).

Finally, in *Desarrollo psíquico. El tiempo y la individuación a lo largo del ciclo vital* (2008), the only work in Spanish, the articles focus on the developmental line of time; one of them specifically refers to midlife, also taking into account the developmental line of acceptance of time limitation and personal death previously mentioned.

Lack of research and contributions by this author (Montero) (2001–2010)

From the first decade of this century onwards, the topic of midlife seems to have lost transcendence, with a reduction in the quantity of books and papers on this theme. Only isolated references have appeared, together with self-help books. However, no consistent effort to go further into the subject seems to have emerged. Nevertheless, during this period this author carried out a series of works that have been presented from 2000 onwards; they could be summed up in various levels.

In 1989, he presented the first paper on midlife: *La travesía por la mitad de la vida* (2005) [The Midlife Journey]. The work gave rise to a research group that resulted in the *Fundación Travesía*, an entity dedicated to the psychoanalytic study of middle age up to this day. The paper could be considered an attempt to describe the different aspects of middle age, in a line of thought still very much influenced by Jaques.

The paper mentioned above was followed by *Las vicisitudes terminables e interminables de la mediana edad* (2000), presented in the Internal Symposium of the APA (Argentine Psychoanalytical Association) as well as in other Congresses during the same year; *Psicoanálisis de la transición y crisis de mediana edad*, presented in different versions at the FEPAL Congress (Montevideo, 2003) and at the CAP (Rosario, 2004). One of the versions was submitted as promotion work for full membership of the APA, published in Trieb magazine (SBPRJ, 2005); it obtained Mention of Honour of the Sebastián Kern 2004 Prize (Porto Alegre). In addition, co-authored *Transience during Midlife as an Adult Psychic Organizer. The Midlife Transition & Crisis Continuum*, written in collaboration with Calvin Anthony Colarusso, presented at the IPA Congress (Rio de Janeiro, 2005) and published in *The Psychoanalytic Study of the Child* (2007). Only some of the papers presented have been mentioned. It must be pointed out that none of these works were focused on the perspective of maturescence.

Furthermore, the work *Psicoanálisis del trauma por la propia muerte futura en la mediana edad* (Montero, 2005a) had a significant impact in the psychoanalytic field, being quoted by various authors, even though this author now considers that the concept presented on that occasion was limiting. In any event, the idea of trauma, which has an anticipatory and continuous effect, precisely because it has not yet occurred, is a very strong metaphor that allows us to assess the magnitude of psychic work involved in maturescence.

With Freud (1914c) as a starting point, this author puts forward a metapsychological concept that evinces the pathognomonic conflict of midlife:

> The most touchy point in the narcissistic system, the immortality of the ego, which is so hard pressed by reality.
>
> (Montero, 2005a) [p. 91]

This reference would be the *external or manifest* metapsychological perspective of his corresponding *internal or latent* one—the source of maturescence—something which he had not conceptualized then.

Further on in *Psicoanálisis del trauma por la propia muerte futura en la mediana edad* (Montero, 2005a), the Freudian concepts integrate themselves with the current proposal:

> Human beings' belonging to nature and the power of *Ananké* (exigencies of life), the latter conceive as the final vital need of dying—something which conscience systematically tries to deny—is another evidence of the constant exposition to the *trauma of one's own future death*. In addition, *Ananké* could mean both the inextricable intimate link with the biological nature of human beings, destined to die, and the impossibility or difficulty of representing one's own death, posed by Freud, which we have already alluded to.
>
> [p. 45]

He then detailed somatic aspects and the kind of work specifically demanded during midlife. The following lines, therefore, function as true precursors of the proposals this author has dealt with in greater depth in later research:

> Universals (invariants and their transformations) of trauma regarding one's own future death, characteristic of midlife, focus mainly on the multiple manifestations of the body. One's own body progressively evinces the anticipated mark of death in the incipient and unmistakable signs of aging and illness, registered as fear of aging and of illness; psychic previews of the reality of the final (definite) trauma of death. This anxiety can also reflect the unconscious perception of certain metabolic, physiological or hormonal (feminine menopause, masculine climacteric) processes.
>
> (Montero, 2005a) [p. 51]

He then suggests considering the ego in the same way Freud (1923b) does:

> The ego is first and foremost a bodily ego.
>
> (Montero, 2005a) [p. 26]

Further on, he proposes:

> From this perspective, the *exigencies of reality* would be represented by the omnipresent, chronic and universal triumph of biology subjugating the anatomical body and the drive body; in the latter case, the anatomical body is invested with libido and aggression, the proper body of psychoanalysis. The different vicissitudes originated by this process have much to do with the fact that, in all of Freud's models of the psychic apparatus, the body is recognized as a real external object whereby the ego maintains an object relationship.
>
> (Montero, 2005a) [p. 68]

This author also considered a few (invariant) universals, which he proposed as the elements to be considered in order to understand the kind of psychic work that midlife demands. At that time, he detailed the (evolution) transformation of narcissism, the actualization of the ego ideal, the reactivation of the pre-oedipal and oedipal conflict and the history of identifications and de-identifications.

Another important milestone with respect to this author's work is the updating of the 2005 paper, previously mentioned, published in *Revista de Psicoanálisis* of the Asociación Psicoanalítica Argentina, with the title *Elementos para una metapsicología de la mediana edad y su relación con la muerte* [Elements for a metapsychology of midlife and its relation with death]. This article introduces an important modification: the key to understanding midlife is centered in the activation of a narcissistic crisis. For this reason, a renewed status is assigned to the transformation of narcissism as the most important invariant, giving it a general and encompassing character that subsumes the categories of the mourning task, together with the other three, in the same order they had been previously formulated.

Thus, the conceptualization that commences with Freud (1930a [1929]) resonates in these Freudian lines quoted by this author:

> We are threatened with suffering from three directions: from our own body, which is doomed to decay and dissolution and which cannot even do without pain and anxiety as warning signals; from the external world, which may rage against us with overwhelming and merciless forces of destruction; and finally from our relations to other men.
>
> (Montero, 2005a) [p. 77]

Significantly, Freud considers that the body—in the *soma* sense—occupies first place with regard to these three threats, in accordance with the present argument.

Somehow, all this period found expression in the book: *La travesía por la mitad de la vida: Exégesis psicoanalítica* (Montero, 2005b).

Other studies

It is also important to point out that, in Argentina, Graciela Zarebski has dealt at length with the aging issue, giving special attention to midlife. Her concept of the anticipation of aging (Zarebski, 1999) as well as the concept of human reserve (2011) implies the acceptance of one's own aging. The author proposes the idea of *pro-age*, in direct opposition to the *anti-age* movements. The most significant contribution is presented in *Cuestionario Mi Envejecer* [My Aging Questionnaire] (2014), a survey that works as an instrument to evaluate the subjective attitude with regard to one's own aging.

Miscellany

There is an overabundance of psychological literature regarding middle age. They could be mentioned Fried (1967), Clay (1984) and Dubrovsky (1985); among the journalistic literature: Sheehy (1976) and Hermann-Schreiber (1977); and religious: Grün (1980). This author would also like to mention the socio-anthropo-psychological compilation works by Smelser and Erikson (1980). Finally, the works of psychoanalytical dissemination by Nichols (1986) and Mizrahi (1987)—it is impossible and unnecessary to mention them all—only highlighting in this case those texts published in Spanish. Among these, it could also be included the book this author co-authored with Alicia Mirta Ciancio (2008): *Para comprender la mediana edad. Historias de Vida.*

Such an abundance of more popular works evinces that midlife is a phenomenon that has been studied from very different perspectives, even if with a methodology stemming from disciplines that often seem to have no direct connection with psychoanalysis.

Perhaps this author could rescue a different work, among so many others. Fried (1967) introduces the concept of *middlescent*, relating the midlife crisis with adolescence. He attaches importance to the hormonal factor, explaining that climacteric comes from the Greek *climakter*, *step in a staircase*, meaning any change of course during a critical period of life. This term was later adopted to refer to the loss of reproductive capacity in general.

Fried's proposal, even though in a more popular style, comes closer to the one proposed with this book, especially when she suggests the link between midlife and adolescence; she maintains that the hormonal factors—somatic factors—are what promote the midlife crisis—psychic factors—as she terms this stage.

Five questions for a survey about midlife (2009)

As a theoretical background, it is interesting to review the work this author undertook in 2009. It consisted of a series of in-depth interviews focused on midlife carried out at the Congress of the International Psychoanalytic Association in Chicago. The interviewees were several recognized psychoanalysts who attended the Congress.

The idea was to request a filmed 50-minute interview that would be later edited in a video. The objective of the interview was to discuss ideas based on a questionnaire that had been previously sent by email. The participants had the freedom to answer as they saw fit. For this reason, some interviewees chose to adhere to the questionnaire layout while others preferred to use the questions as background for a theorization which did not spare improvisations or personal confessions.

Of course, the selection of colleagues as interviewees can be criticized. Nevertheless, it is still a partial sample of psychoanalysis, considering that the participants were conspicuous members of the IPA world, because the interviewed colleagues did not form part of the rest of the psychoanalytic world.

After the editing of the original video, several colleagues who had participated suggested a textual transcription of each interview and a revision on the part of each interviewee, with the purpose of an eventual production in book form. This resulted in the book entitled *Updating Midlife: Psychoanalytic Perspectives* (Montero et al., 2013).

The questionnaire sent by email included the following questions:

1.1 Do you consider there is such a thing as *midlife* and would it be appropriate to talk about *midlife*?
1.2 How would you define midlife?
1.3 Do you think that there is a specificity regarding midlife equivalent to what psychoanalysis grants to adolescence? If so, do you consider midlife as a developmental phase?
2.1 Which specifically theoretical concepts posed by Freud do you consider useful for an understanding of midlife? What is more, how would you explain midlife in the light of Freud's theories and concepts?
3.1 How would you define the general and metapsychological characteristics of midlife from your own theoretical framework?
3.2 What happens during midlife? What would you consider its the psychological landscape?
3.3 When does the onset of midlife occur? What main paths does midlife go through?
4.1 What questions and answers would you like to add to this midlife questionnaire?
5.1 Please feel free to include here any topic of interest, not necessarily related to midlife.

The professionals invited to participate were: Dr Alcira Mariam Alizade (Buenos Aires), Christopher Bollas MD (England), Dott Stefano Bolognini (Italy), Calvin Anthony Colarusso MD (USA), Dott Franco de Masi (Italy), Dr Cláudio Laks Eizirik (Brazil), Dr Haydée Faimberg (France), Glen O. Gabbard MD (USA), Charles M T Hanly MD (Canada), Dr Luis Kancyper (Argentina), Dr Norberto Carlos Marucco (Argentina), Leo Rangell MD (USA) and Dr David Rosenfeld (Argentina). Of course, the video and later book also included this author's considerations.

The wealth of answers did not necessarily include the somatic source that promotes drive increase, but the result of the interviews made it possible to put together a scheme that enables the reader to perceive how midlife was being considered.

Now an attempt to summarize each author's thoughts, with the exception of Colarusso and de Masi, whose concepts have already been considered. The result of the series of interviews was dissimilar with this author's views, since many of the psychoanalytic tenets clearly concealed the latent contents of mid-life—indirect comprehension of maturescence.

Alizade's contributions focused on the differentiation between the healthy and the pathological as well as his concepts of what is positive in psychoanalysis and tertiary narcissism, which he elaborated in a chapter, once his personal interview had been filmed:

> Becoming conscious of midlife may produce either healthy or pathological transformations. Amongst the healthy ones we find: narcissism transformation, detachment, the work of consciousness, an increase of intelligence and maturational processes, the working-through of impermanence, and a wider view of the world (greater reality principle). The pathological transformations encompass: horror of old age, fear of death, pathological attachment and fear of abandonment.
>
> (Montero et al., 2013) [p. 3]

> As long as consciousness can control the unconscious narcissistic system that claims for the ego's immortality (Freud, 1914c), dying will not be a tragedy. This faculty requires the transformation of narcissism towards a type of narcissism that I posed as tertiary narcissism. It could also be named *beyond narcissism*. This sort of narcissism overcomes the interaction between ego libido and object libido. The narcissistic circle gradually opens up and the individual places narcissism out of himself. His libidinal interest expands and narcissism turns towards exogamy, towards others, people he will never meet although they become a source of interest (far-off objects). Feelings and actions of solidarity could also appear through generational transference.
>
> (Montero et al., 2013) [p. 5]

Christopher Bollas dedicated his interview to an expressive freedom game and an apparent improvisation. Some of his most relevant paragraphs are here:

> I think this is the prevailing question of midlife: Who am I? If the question during adolescence is: What am I becoming?, the question of young adulthood might be, at twenty-five or twenty-seven years of age: Where do I come from, who were my parents, my father, my mother?; then, I think the question in the mid-thirties or mid-forties is: Who am I? and the question in the middle-sixties is: What was this all about, what was life all about?
>
> (Montero et al., 2013) [p. 11]

> There is something related to the genuine uniformity of the human body. We talked about the impact of midlife, but in late adulthood there are life-threatening changes to life itself. Death is close by, and of course, we have always known this, but in our attempt to prepare ourselves for death, through reading, through philosophical discussion, I could say that nothing that can prepare us for the encounter with the real in its manifestations. As Lacan said, the embodiment of the real is death itself. So, I think there is something, that leads me to feel very fond of people of my age, I am very happy to see people of my age, much more than when I was middle aged. I really think there is something heroic in being human, let's call it the struggle of being human. There is something heroic about this. Because I think that the people I admire have accepted their mortality, I think you can feel it, and there is nothing morbid about it, not even a manic state of denial, etc. It's very moving, and there is a different temporality in old age, because until the middle sixties, more or less, we can look at the age of thirty, thirty-five, forty, and we can see them as sorts of markers of the chronology of life, but when we get to our sixties, chronology no longer means anything. I don't think that sixty-five, seventy, or seventy-five mean much anymore, you know, because the time that moves forward no longer does so in the same manner nor does it have the same celebratory meaning. So there is a kind of timelessness, a late temporality that we arrive at in old age. We have therefore intriguing dimensions in common with unconscious life itself, I think we come closer to oneiric life in old age than ever before, and that our dreams have greater resonance and wisdom; we listen to them much more, we pay more attention to them. This is the intensity of old age and we want to continue being alive.
>
> (Montero et al., 2013) [p. 22]

Stefano Bolognini maintains:

> There is a specificity during this period, and this specificity is given by an increased awareness of our place in the community, our place in life, our responsibility, and also the acknowledgement that the community gives to

a man or a woman who has developed something good in his or her life. That is why it [midlife] is a strange, rich period, where achievements are recognized when there is a reason for doing so, but at the same time, the limit is perceived much more clearly than before.

(Montero et al., 2013) [p. 26]

Cláudio Laks Eizirik emphasizes the importance of generational transference:

I think there is a progressive notion that the things we do will be our way of surviving. I would say that our main creation are our children or our students, the disciples. But our children and grandchildren are within the concept of generativity referred to by Erikson, but in the sense of art, or artistic creation. There are simple examples of this, not necessarily from great artists but, for instance, from a grandmother who teaches her granddaughter the recipes she had learnt from her mother; or a father who teaches his son how to play football or fly a kite; small things from everyday life that express something artistic and, maybe, are a way of continuing to live. Thus, we might have the opportunity of listening to a child or a grandchild saying something we had told him many years ago but we had forgotten.

(Montero et al., 2013) [p. 70]

Haydée Faimberg did not accept the filmed interview but she agreed to write a chapter for the book. In it she finds her own concept of midlife, developing her concept of a *telescoping of generations*:

The recognition of otherness (or what the other *is* and *desires*) and of the difference between generations is a momentous step which marks the transition from a narcissistic to an Oedipal mode of functioning. I consider that the *alienating, unconscious narcissistic identifications* where always there, and a *telescoping of three generations* can be found in all advanced analysis (Faimberg, 2005). If we have worked this issue analytically and in depth, there is a likelihood that the process of giving, once again, a new retroactive meaning to the relation between generations and the recognition of otherness will be reactivated when the patient becomes a parent (or a training analyst). I am leaving aside other ways in which this process may be triggered.

(Montero et al., 2013) [p. 86]

Glen O. Gabbard maintains:

It can occur anywhere from the age of thirty-five up to the fifties, although now with people who are living productively into their eighties, numerical boundaries are different and perhaps it could now begin a bit later. But the point, I think, is when the individual comes to recognize the limits of his omnipotence, that life will not go on forever, that there is a body that is aging, and a health that is deteriorating, and, of course, the existential themes of death, mourning and meaning.

(Montero et al., 2013) [p. 94]

Asked about the metapsychology of midlife, Gabbard described it as follows:

Relevant metapsychology involves a working-through of the depressive position, as I mentioned earlier, and often the onset is related to some sense of loss and guilt. For example, a parent dies, and one thinks: I should have been a better son or daughter, I wish I had done more for my mother or father. This is sobering awareness of one's own narcissism and one's capacity to hurt and neglect those one loves.

(Montero et al., 2013) [p. 96]

Charles M. T. Hanly, invited to participate in the project due to his concept of ideal of the ego and ego ideal, sustains:

I would define the threshold and the central struggle of midlife as a kind of narcissistic anxiety, a threat to the loss of self-esteem, consequent upon the unequivocal and inescapable realization that nature does not estimate or esteem us as we estimate and esteem ourselves. We are confronted with, and discover, what has always been there for us to know but we have only known with a passing glance over our shoulder, our temporal finitude. There are numerous other variable factors from individual to individual, but I take this factor to be the essential cause of the midlife crisis that everyone experiences to some extent. How it is dealt with by the individual is a crucial factor in the way in which people live their midlife and prepare themselves for old age.

(Montero et al., 2013) [p. 104]

Hanly suggests that the causes of the typical midlife crisis are the following:

Another, yet more tragic, failure occurs when the quantity of parental object love for the young is replaced by a narcissistic identification with young people. Middle-aged people begin to behave as if they were still teenagers in a doomed effort of reincarnation by imitation. An example is the accountant who trades in the family SUV for a Harley-Davidson, lets what is left of his hear grow long, and suits himself out in teenage grubs for the iconic cross-country tour. Another is the lawyer who abandons his wife of many years for a younger woman. There is a risk of an enacted regression in midlife that can be very damaging and tragic for the individual and for his or her family. This more severe regression evinces the failure of midlife as it reactivates dormant conflicts, in so far as one of its great tasks is the preparation for old age.

(Montero et al., 2013) [p. 107]

Luis Kancyper, for his part, maintains:

> I would say that midlife is a cam stage in contrast with adolescence or old age. At this moment silent mourning processes take place throughout all the structures: narcissistic, Oedipal, and fraternal structures. There are also gradual and silent changes in the body including fertility, which puts a limit to immortality. By being fertile, I not only mean having a child but also a social position, having a house, money, or some work of our own. By the way, advertisements for employment also make a point when asking for people up to forty or forty-five years old. They are indicating the age of power but within a boundary. On account of fertility–infertility, I would like to point out that it is not about being sterile but being fertile in its widest range of meanings.
>
> (Montero et al., 2013) [p. 114]

Norberto Carlos Marucco emphasizes the structuring mechanism of denial of psychic life:

> Although there is a pathological denial, there is also a general denial which borders normal psychic mechanisms. For instance, the denial of reality that naturally takes place in adolescence and triggers development during this stage of life. Interestingly, in midlife a natural balance occurs between accepting and denying reality. What do I mean by this? It is a period of life where some wishes could have been fulfilled, but others have not; and these latter ones that couldn't be fulfilled can be acknowledged and sublimated. I believe that midlife is the most important moment in life for sublimatory phenomena, due to this mechanism of acknowledging and denying reality, acknowledging what will be achieved and what will never be accomplished.
>
> (Montero et al., 2013) [p. 120]

Leo Rangell, attempts to define midlife crisis:

> What I think causes a midlife crisis, somewhere between forty and fifty, is that this is usually the crucial time for an assessment of the second half of one's life. I think that a disturbance in that period, in that decade, can occur if there is a sudden and abrupt dissatisfaction caused by a disruption experienced either in love, work, or friendships. Where these three lines of interrelationships have been satisfactory, and promise to continue bringing comfort, pleasure, and enjoyment, one can settle down peacefully without any concern. But when there is a sudden change in direction towards a dissatisfaction coming from any one of those three great areas, a disturbance of love, a break in satisfaction with one's mate, or a sudden loss of work success, this may initiate an emotional feeling that changes the course of life's trajectory from one of increasing satisfaction to one of

doubt and worries about whether or not satisfaction will continue. If one feels that what lies ahead is not likely to produce the same comfort level as the first half of life, anxiety intervenes and a decline may set in.

(Montero et al., 2013) [p. 150]

Finally, David Rosenfeld, views the concept of midlife from a completely different perspective:

At a psychological level (according to Jean Paul Sartre's philosophical analysis), midlife does not exist as a "thing-in-itself." Neither does *acting-out* exist as a *thing-in-itself*. It is a definition used by psychoanalysts to describe certain behaviors. The same would apply for the midlife concept: it is something defined by the analyst in his field of work. It is not something that exists on its own; it is a very interesting concept, but it should not be formulated in the abstract. We could talk about midlife or middle-age from two different angles: biologically or as a psychological concept. The latter would consider a patient's midlife when he is capable of introspection, insight, and he can realize that he has come a long way in life and still has half of his life left to live.

(Montero et al., 2013) [p. 157]

The immense wealth and great capacity to understand psychological phenomena reflected in each interview evinces that those who participated in the project did so taking into account not only their own clinical work but also their life experience. Be this as it may, this author must highlight that the metapsychological key used lies in Freud's (1914c) words, as has been already pointed out:

The most touchy point in the narcissistic system, the immortality of the ego, which is so hard pressed by reality.

(Montero et al., 2013) [p. 91]

Perhaps this premise was what prevented the key theme of maturescence from emerging as it is understood nowadays.

Research by this author (Montero) (2011–2020)

This author will maintain references to a minimum, since from 2013 they have been integrated to his elaboration of maturescence, detailed in this book. It would be therefore mentioned: *Enfrentando el dolor por la madurescencia. Definición, metapsicología y clínica*, which appeared in Revista de Psicoanálisis de la Asociación Psicoanalítica Argentina (2013); *Psychoanalysis of Maturescence (Definition, Metapsychology and Clinical Practice)*, published in *The International Journal of Psychoanalysis* (2015); and *La disrupción somático-instintiva (peri)climatérica como un factor del incremento pulsional madurescente*, Doctoral Thesis presented at the Universidad del Salvador, in agreement with the Argentine Psychoanalytic Association.

Current non-psychoanalytic research

It has not been easy to find research currently undertaken on the topic of mid-life and its link with the perspective of maturescence. Nevertheless, we were able to acquaint ourselves with two important studies. The first one, by Orville Gilbert Brim MD, and he second, a well-publicized study of the "U" curve in human emotional life by Andrew Oswald and David Blanchflower (2008).

In addition, Brim (2004) leads an ongoing and far-reaching research. He carried out a study in the United States, sponsored by the MacArthur Foundation, to determine the degree of satisfaction with life of persons during midlife. These investigations are becoming available by a series of papers, each one detailing different sub-items as the years go by. The notebooks and interviews each participant had to respond to and undergo, which were truly comprehensive, have been followed over the course of decades. The MIDI (*Midlife Development Inventory*), is so comprehensive that it includes all biomedical data, family ties, social and economic background, etc., all divided into sections. This research continues in the United Sates and has included 8,000 subjects which have participated in the study for many decades.

Even though the above study is very comprehensive, the somatic data requested to the participants are only provided statistically, since they aim at a factual rather than a subjective understanding. The reason for this could be that the purpose of the investigation by the MacArthur Foundation does not entail a psychoanalytical understanding or even a psychological one of the causes of satisfaction or dissatisfaction in midlife. Instead, it aims at an understanding that integrates such variables as: psychological, sociological, economic, anthropological, etc., attempting to measure the satisfaction with life from a different perspective.

On the other hand, Blanchflower and Oswald (2008), MIT economists, carried out research that crossed data from 80 countries, analyzing the emotional state and satisfaction with life of thousands of people from 35 to 70 years of age. Their results indicated a "U" curve, where the lowest part coincided with what has been termed midlife crisis, with the nadir at 45 years of age. They concluded that whether the subjects had had children or not, were married or divorced, or had experienced economic success, etc., a general depression appears in the population as a whole. This could be expressed as a dissatisfaction, among many other symptoms, which tends to decrease at 50 years of age, finally stabilizing towards satisfaction around 60 years of age.

It should be stressed that the researchers are economists who obtained psychological conclusions using variables that would be difficult to transfer to the methodology used by psychoanalysis. Moreover, regardless of the study's transcendence, certain researchers question its statistic validity, since it does not consider variables that could represent a true empirical study. Nevertheless, the large degree of publicity obtained by the investigation brought midlife to the forefront once again. Furthermore, the concept of the "U" curve has been repeated as something established in relevant journals and congresses, with the risk of adopting it as a generalization that avoids, once again, taking individual variables and their processing into account as well as *a direct comprehension of maturescence*, as this book tries to highlight. Of course, even though it was not possible to have access to the data, it could be considered that, in part, the results obtained by Blanchflower and Oswald (2008) coincided with this proposal, since drive increase associated with climacterics upon the background of underlying aphanisis, could be experienced as dissatisfaction, depression, anxiety. etc.

In addition, this author would like to mention Jonathan Rauch's article, published in *The Atlantic* in December, 2014. The magazine dedicates seven pages in color to the topic of midlife, based on the "U" curve of happiness; the article takes for granted that this theory is a universal that occurs to everyone. The journalist suggests considering how contemporary science managed to find a correlation between aging and happiness by means of the "U" curve. The price of publicity, of course, is that we must endure the stereotypes attached to the social representation of midlife. An example of this is the magazine's cover depicting a middle-aged man in a red convertible, with a sad expression and sunglasses on his forehead. The perspective of this book is miles away from this image because midlife, and specifically the maturescent process, could be precisely the opportunity for a change rather than the regression suggested by the image.

Finally, this author would like to stress that both studies aim at the welfare and satisfaction that take place around midlife. However, they seem consider this wellbeing as something that appears in advance, rather than as the result of a working-through of drive increase confronted with the background of the underlying aphanisis and the multiple variables that include the life history and subjectivity of an individual. Furthermore, they do not seem to consider the psychic processes, but only take into account external affective manifestations.

Bibliography

Index of references

1. Works by Sigmund Freud
2. Psychoanalytic and Psychological Works
3. Other Works
4. Works by Guillermo Julio Montero

I. Works by Sigmund Freud

Freud, S. (1900a). *The Interpretation of Dreams*. The Standard Edition, Volumes 4 and 5.

Freud, S. (1904a [1904]) *On Psychotherapy*. Volume 7.

Freud, S. (1905e [1901]). *Fragment of an Analysis of a Case of Hysteria*. Volume 7.

Freud, S. (1909c [1908]). *Family Romances*. Volume 9.

Freud, S. (1910c). *Leonardo da Vinci and a Memory of his Childhood*. Volume 11.

Freud, S. (1911b). *Formulations on the Two Principles of Mental Functioning*. Volume 12.

Freud, S. (1912–1913). *Totem and Taboo*. Volume 13.

Freud, S. (1912c). *Types of Onset of Neurosis*. Volume 12.

Freud, S. (1912f). *Contributions to a Discussion on Masturbation*. Volume 12.

Freud, S. (1914c). *On Narcissism: An Introduction*. Volume 14.

Freud, S. (1915a). *Instincts and Their Vicissitudes*. Volume 14.

Freud, S. (1915b). *Thoughts for the Times of War and Death*. Volume 14.

Freud, S. (1915c). *Instincts and Their Vicissitudes*. Volume 14.

Freud, S. (1916–1917 [1915–1917]). *Introductory Lectures on Psychoanalysis*. Volume 16.

Freud, S. (1916a [1915]). *On Transience*. Volume 14.

Freud, S. (1916d). *Some Character Types Met with in Psycho-Analytic Work*. Volume 14.

Freud, S. (1917a). *A Difficulty in the Path of Psycho-Analysis*. Volume 17.

Freud, S. (1917e [1915]). *Mourning and Melancholia*. Volume 14.

Freud, S. (1919a [1918]). *Lines of Advance in Psycho-Analytic Therapy*. Volume 17.

Freud, S. (1919h). *The Uncanny*. Volume 17.

Freud, S. (1920g). *Beyond the Pleasure Principle*. Volume 18.

Freud, S. (1921). *Group Psychology and the Analysis of the Ego*. Volume 18.

Freud, S. (1921c). *Group Psychology and the Analysis of the Ego*. Volume 18.

Freud, S. (1923b). *The Ego and the Id*. Volume 19.

Freud, S. (1924e). *The Loss of Reality in Neurosis and Psychosis*. Volume 19.

Freud, S. (1926d [1925]). *Inhibitions, Symptoms and Anxiety*. Volume 20.

Freud, S. (1926e). *The Question of Lay Analysis*. Volume 20.

Freud, S. (1927c). *The Future of an Illusion*. Volume 21.

Freud, S. (1930a [1929]). *Civilization and its Discontents*. Volume 21.

Freud, S. (1931d). *The Expert Opinion in the Halsmann Case*. Volume 21.

Freud, S. (1933a [1932]). *New Introductory Lectures on Psycho-Analysis*. Volume 22.

Freud, S. (1937c). *Analysis Terminable and Interminable*. Volume 23.

Freud, S. (1940a [1938]). *An Outline of Psycho-Analysis*. Volume 23.

Freud, S. (1940b [1938]). *Some Elementary Lessons in Psycho-Analysis*. Volume 23.

Freud, S. (1950a [1887–1902]). *Project for a Scientific Psychology*. Volume 1.

Strachey, J. (ed.. y Trad.) *The Standard Edition of the Complete Psychological Works of Sigmund Freud*. The Hogarth Press, London.

2. Psychoanalytic and Psychological Works

Anzieu, D. (1986). *Freud's Self-Analysis*. The International Psycho-Analytical Library, The Hogarth Press, London.

Baranger, W. (1961). *La situación analítica como campo dinámico*. Revista Uruguaya de Psicoanálisis, Montevideo.

Bergler, E. (1954). *The Revolt of the Middle-Aged Man*. Grosset and Dunlap, New York.

Bion, W.R.B. (1962). *Learning from Experience*. Jason Aronson, London.

Bion, W.R.B. (1990). *Two Papers. The Grid and Caesura*. Karnac Books, London.

Blanchflower, D. & Oswald, A. (2008). *Is Well-Being U-Shaped over the Life Cycle?* Department of Economics, Darthmouth.

Blos, P. (1979). *The Adolescent Passage. Developmental Issues*. Intrnational Universities Press, New York.

Bollas, C. (1989). *Forces of Destiny: Psychoanalysis and Human Idiom*. Free Associations, London.

Brim, O.G. (2004). *How Healthy Are We?: A National Study of Well-Being at Midlife (The John D. And Catherine T. MacArthur Foundation Series)*. The University of Chicago Press, Chicago, IL.

Ciancio, A.M. (2014): *Personal Communication*. FEPAL Psychoanalytic Congress, Buenos Aires.

Clay, J. (1984). *El hombre más allá de los 40. Sus esperanzas, sus emociones, sus proyectos*. Paidós, Barcelona, 1992.

Colarusso, C.A. & Nemiroff, R.A. (1981). *Adult Development: A New Dimension in Psychodynamic Theory and Practice*. Plenum Press, New York.

Colarusso, C.A. & Nemiroff, R.A. (1985). *The Race Against Time: Psychoanalysis and Psychotherapy in the Second Half of Life*. Plenum Press, New York.

Colarusso, C.A. & Nemiroff, R.A. (eds.) (1990). *New Dimensions in Adult Development*. Basic Books, New York.

Colarusso, C.A. (1992). *Child and Adult Development: A Psychodynamic Introduction for Clinicians*. Plenum Press, New York.

Colarusso, C.A. (1994). *Fulfillment in Adulthood: Paths to the Pinnacle of Life*. Plenum Press, New York.

Colarusso, C.A. (1999). The Development of Time Sense in Middle Adulthood. *The Psychoanalytic Quarterly*, volume 68.

Colarusso, C.A. (2000). Separation–Individuation Phenomena in Adulthood: General Concepts and the Fifth Individuation. *Journal of the American Psychoanalytic Association*, volume 48.

Colarusso, C.A. (2008). *Desarrollo psíquico: El tiempo y la individuación a lo largo del ciclo vital*. Entrevía, Buenos Aires.

de Masi, F. (2002). *Making Death Thinkable. Psychoanalytic Contribution to the Problem on the Transience of Life*. Free Association, New York.

Dubrovsky, S. (1985). *Crisis de vida en la mediana edad (35–55 años)*. Galerna, Buenos Aires, 1985.

Erikson, E. (1951). *Childhood and Society*. Norton, New York.

Faimberg, H. (2005). *The Telescoping of Generations: Listening to the Narcissistic Links Between Generations*. Routledge, London.

Freud, A. (1963). The Concept of Developmental Lines. *The Psychoanalytic Study of the Child*, volume 18.

Freud, A. *et al*. (1965). Metapsychological Assessment of the Adult Personality: The Adult Profile. *The Psychoanalytic Study of the Child*, volume 20.

Freud, S. (1937). *Letter to Marie Bonaparte*. PEP Archives.

Freud, S. (1985). *The Complete Letters of Sigmund Freud to Wilhelm Fliess 1887–1904*. The Belknap Press, Harvard University Press, Cambridge.

Fried, B. (1967). *Para una madurez sin crisis*. La Aurora, Buenos Aires, 1983.

Greenspan, S.I. & Pollock, G.H. (1980). *The Course of Life: Psychoanalytic Contributions Toward Understanding Personality Development*. Maryland Menthal Health Study Center, Maryland.

Grün, A. (1980). *La mitad de la vida como tarea espiritual. La crisis de los 40–50 años*. Narcea, Madrid, 1988.

Hanly, C. (1983). Ego Ideal and Ideal Ego. *The International Journal of Psycho-Analysis*, Volume 65, 1984.

Herman-Schreiber, J.J. (1977). *La crisis de la mediana edad*. Huemul, Buenos Aires, 1978.

Jacobi, J. (1939): *The Psychology of C. G. Jung*, Routledge, London.

Jaques, E. (1965). Death and the Mid-Life Crisis. *International Journal of Psycho-Analysis*, Volume 46, pp. 502–514.

Jones, E. (1927). The Early Development of Female Sexuality. *The International Jornal of Psychoanalysis*, Volume 8, pp. 459–472.

Jones, E. (1955). *Sigmund Freud: Life and Work, Volume Two: Years of Maturity 1901–1919*, The Hogarth Press, London.

Jung, C.G. (1930). *The Stages of Life. Collected Works*, Volume 8, Princeton University Press, Princeton.

Kavka, A. (2014). *Panel: Psychoanalytic Perspectives on Aging's Committee*, FEPAL Congress, Buenos Aires.

Kernberg, O. (1980). *Internal World and External Reality: Object Relations Theory Applied*. Jason Aronson, Northvale.

King, P. (1980). The Life Cycle as Indicated by the Nature of the Transference in the Psychoanalysis of the Middle-Aged and Elderly. *The International Journal of Psychoanalysis*, Volume 61, pp. 153–160.

Klein, M. (1963). On the Sense of Loneliness. In: *Envy and Gratitude and Other Works*. New York, The Free Press.

Levinson, D.J. (1978). *The Season's of a Man's Life*. Random House, New York.

Levinson, D.J. (1996). *The Season's of a Woman's Life*. Alfred Knopf, New York.

Mahler, M.S. (1968). *On Human Symbiosis and the Vicissitudes of Individuation*. International Universities Press, New York.

Mahler, M.S. (1977). Developmental Aspects in the Assessment of Narcissistic and So-Called Borderline Patients. In: *Selected Papers of Margaret Mahler*, volume 2. Jason Aronson, Northvale.

Mizrahi, L. (1987). *La mujer transgresora*. Grupo Editor Latinoamericano, Buenos Aires.

Neugarten, B.L. (1996). *The meanings of Age: Selected Papers of Bernice L. Neugarten*. The University of Chicago Press, Chicago, IL.

Nichols, M.P. (1986). *Análisis psicológico de la crisis a los cuarenta años relacionada con los cambios en la década actual*. Gedisa, Barcelona, 1987.

Rauch, J. (2014). *The Real Roots of Midlife Crisis*. The Atlantic.

Schur, M. (1972). *Freud: Living and Dying*. International Universities Press, New York.

Segal, H. (1984). Joseph Conrad and the Midlife Crisis. In: *Psychoanalysis, Literature and War*. New Library of Psychoanalysis, London.

Sheehy, G. (1976). *Passages*. Ballantine Books, New York.

Singman de Vogelfanger, L. (2006). La función adulta en la confrontación generacional. De la claudicación a la continuidad. In: *Mediana edad: Estudios psicoanalíticos*. Entrevía, Buenos Aires.

Smelser, N.J. & Erikson, E. (1980). *Trabajo y amor en la edad adulta*. Grijalbo, Barcelona, 1982.

Spitz, R.A. (1965). *The First Year of Life*.International Universities Press, New York.

Stein, M. (1983): *In Midlife: A Jungian Perspective*. Spring Publications, Dallas.

Waddell, M. (1998). *Inside Lives. Psychoanalysis and the Growth of the Personality*. Tavistock Clinic Series, London.

Winnicott, D.W. (1971). *Playing and Reality*. Routledge Classics, London.

Zarebski, G. (1999). *Hacia un buen envejecer*. Emecé, Buenos Aires.

Zarebski, G. (2011). *El futuro se construye hoy. La reserva humana*. Paidós, Buenos Aires.

Zarebski, G. (2014). *CME Cuestionario Mi Envejecer. Un instrumento psicogerontológico para evaluar la actitud frente al propio envejecimiento*. Paidos, Buenos Aires.

3. Other works

Barthes, R. (1980). *Camera Lucida. Reflections on Photography*. Hill and Wang, New York.

Cervantes, M. (2005). *Don Quixote*. Ecco Press, New York.

Cave, C. & Oxenham, M. (2017). Sex and the Elderly: Attitudes to long-lived women and men in early Anglo-Saxon England. *Journal of Anthropological Archaeology*, Volume 48, pp. 207–216.

Critchley, S. (2009). *The Book of Dead Philosophers*. Vintage Books, New York.

Damrosch, D. (2006). *The Buried Book. The Loss and Rediscovery of the Great Epic of Gilgamesh*. Holt, New York.

Dawkins, R. (1976). *The Selfish Gene*. Oxford University Press, Oxford.

Descartes, R. (1999). *Meditations and Other Metaphysical Writings*. Penguin Classics, London.

Diamond, J. (1992). *The Third Chimpanzee*. Harper Collins, New York.

Diamond, J. (1997). *Why Is Sex Fun?* Basic Books, New York.

Finley, J.H. (1967). The Heroic Mind. In: *The Odyssey*. Norton Critical Edition, New York, 350–355.

García Gual, C. (1981). *Mitos, viajes, héroes*. Taurus, Madrid.

García Gual, C. (2012). *Enigmático Edipo. Mito y tragedia*. Fondo de Cultura Económica, Madrid.

Gardner, J. & Maier, J. (1984). *Gilgamesh*. Vintage Books, New York.

Goux, J.J. (1999). *Edipo filósofo*. Biblos, Buenos Aires.

Johnson, S. (2009). *The Major Works*. Oxford University Press, Oxford.

McLuhan, M.Y. & Powers, B.R. (1962). *The Gutenberg Galaxy*. University of Toronto Press, Toronto, 2017.

Nabokov, V. (1955). *The Annotated Lolita*. Penguin Books, London, 2000.

Oxford English Reference Dictionary. (1995). Oxford University Press, Oxford.

Petchers, L. (2013). *The Midlife Project*. Documentary at www.vimeo.com

Rawson, H. (1995). *Dictionary of Euphemisms and Other Double-talk*. Crown Publishers, New York.

Said, E (2006). *On Late Style: Music and Literature against the Grain*. Vintage Books, New York.

Shakespeare, W. (2005). *Othello (The Annotated Shakespeare)*. Yale University Press, Yale.

Thomas, D. (2017). *The Poems of Dylan Thomas*. New Directions, New York.

Vernant, J.P. (1996a). Death with Two Faces. In: *Reading The Odyssey*. Princeton University Press, Princeton, 55–61.

Vernant, J.P. (1996b). The Refusal of Oddyseus. In: *Reading The Odyssey*. Princeton University Press, Princeton, 185–189.

Webster's New Universal Unabridged Dictionary. (1996). Barnes & Noble Books, New York.

Woolf, V. (2000). *Mrs Dalloway*. Penguin Modern Classics, London.

Yankélévitch, V. (1977). *La mort*. Flammarion, París.

4. Works by Guillermo Julio Montero

Montero, G.J. (2000). *Las vicisitudes terminables e interminables de la mediana edad*. APA's Symposium & Congreso Interno.

Montero, G.J. (2003). *Psicoanálisis de la transición y crisis de mediana edad*. FEPAL Congress, Montevideo.

Montero, G.J. (2005a). *Psicoanálisis del trauma por la propia muerte futura*. IPA Congress, Rio de Janeiro.

Montero, G.J. (2005b). *La travesía por la mitad de la vida: Exégesis psicoanalítica*. Sapiens, H. Editores, Rosario.

Montero, G.J. (2013). Enfrentando el dolor por la madurescencia. Definición, metapsicología y clínica. *Revista de Psicoanálisis, Asociación Psicoanalítica Argentina*, Volume LXX, number 1.

Montero, G.J. (2015). Psychoanalysis of Maturescence (Definition, Metapsychology and Clinical Practice). *The International Journal of Psychoanalysis*, volume 96, pp. 1491–1513.

Montero, G.J. (2016). *La disrupción somático-instintiva (peri)climatérica como un factor del incremento pulsional madurescente*. PhD Thesis delivered at Universidad del Salvador, Buenos Aires.

Montero, G.J. & Colarusso, C.A. (2007). Transience during Midlife as an Adult Psychic Organizer. The Midlife Transition & Crisis Continuum. *The Psychoanalytic Study of the Child*, volume 62.

Montero, G.J. & Ciancio de Montero, A.M. (2008). *Para comprender la mediana edad. Historias de vida*. Entrevía, Buenos Aires.

Montero, G.J., Ciancio de Montero, A.M. & Singman de Vogelfanger, L. (eds.) (2013). *Updating Midlife: Psychoanalytic Perspectives*. Karnac Books, London.

Index

For Product Safety Concerns and Information please contact our EU
representative GPSR@taylorandfrancis.com
Taylor & Francis Verlag GmbH, Kaufingerstraße 24, 80331 München, Germany